PREGNANCY AND INFANTS: MEDICAL, PSYCHOLOGICAL
AND SOCIAL ISSUES

PREGNANCY AND INFANTS: MEDICAL ISSUES, DISEASES AND HEALTH

PREGNANCY AND INFANTS: MEDICAL, PSYCHOLOGICAL AND SOCIAL ISSUES

Additional books in this series can be found on Nova's website
under the Series tab.

Additional E-books in this series can be found on Nova's website
under the E-books tab.

PREGNANCY AND INFANTS: MEDICAL ISSUES, DISEASES AND HEALTH

TSISANA SHARTAVA
EDITOR

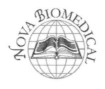

Nova Science Publishers, Inc.

New York

Copyright © 2011 by Nova Science Publishers, Inc.

For permission to use material from this book please contact us:
Telephone 631-231-7269; Fax 631-231-8175
Web Site: http://www.novapublishers.com

NOTICE TO THE READER

LIBRARY OF CONGRESS CATALOGING-IN-PUBLICATION DATA

Pregnancy and infants: medical issues, diseases and health / Tsisana Shartava.
p. cm.
"International Journal Of Medical And Biological Frontiers Volume 16, Issue 1/2."
Includes bibliographical references and index.
ISBN 978-1-61209-132-7 (softcover : alk. paper)
1. Pregnancy. 2. Infants. I. Shartava, Tsisana.
RG551.P737 2011
618.2--dc22
2010047083

Published by Nova Science Publishers, Inc. † New York

CONTENTS

PREFACE

This book presents research done surrounding prevalent medical issues and diseases which pose potential health risks to pregnant women and infants. Topics discussed include multiple sclerosis and appendicitis during pregnancy; probiotics in maternal and early infant nutrition; the treatment of procedural pain in neonates and breastfeeding during crises and emergencies. (Imprint: Nova Biomedical.

Chapter 1 - Multiple sclerosis (MS) is more prevalent in women of childbearing age, posing an extra challenge in the management of this chronic neurological disease. For several decades, women with MS were discouraged from having children, until knowledge accumulated after the work of Confravreux *et al* showed otherwise. In fact, current knowledge shows that the gestational period has a beneficial role in MS relapse rate without affecting the long-term progress of the disease. Additionally, the recent therapeutic advances may help MS women to remain active for a long period of time, providing proper maternal care. However, the relative lack of data from different countries and institutions, as well as the poor information on exposure to MS drugs, create the need for further research on the subject. It is unlikely that any trial on current approved MS drugs will ever consider including pregnant women in the study. Therefore, this chapter summarizes literature data on the MS and pregnancy, discussing the effects of one condition onto the other, and reproductive risks for both mother and child. Many subsections of this chapter are based upon general concepts and several authors' personal opinions, since no evidence-based is available for some questions. Some symptoms of MS may determine different approaches to particular problems, without any evidence-based data. For example, spasticity of lower limbs may affect normal delivery and require cesarean intervention, as discussed forthwith. Other relevant issues of MS symptoms in pregnancy are also discussed along the chapter.

Chapter 2 - Celiac disease, i.e. permanent intolerance to gluten, has an autoimmune mechanism. Controversy exists in the literature regarding the association between celiac and infertility, abortions, intra-uterine growth restriction (IUGR) and stillbirths. When properly managed, celiac disease might have little effect on pregnancy and birth outcomes. However, as a commonly undiagnosed disease, fertility, pregnancy, and birth might all be negatively affected by it when it is unrecognized and untreated. When celiac disease is untreated, women may be subfertile, or suffer infertility. If a woman manages to become pregnant without treating celiac disease, there are higher rates of IUGR, and low birthweight (LBW) of her offspring. Therefore, celiac disease should be considered among idiopathic infertility repeat spontaneous abortion, and immediately and strictly treated in order to correct future risks. Control of a gluten-free diet is important in terms of healthy reproduction. Further, studies should focus on screening for celiac disease among patients presenting with IUGR of an unknown etiology.

Chapter 3 - The incidence of appendicitis during pregnancy is equal to that in the normal population. However, during pregnancy appendicitis may occur with a variety of clinical presentations, thereby causing severe diagnostic difficulties, especially during the second half of gestation. As a result, appendicitis during pregnancy is associated with an increase in perforation rate, morbidity and mortality compared to that in the normal population. In addition, it may cause pre-term birth and/or fetal loss.

In this chapter we review diagnostic and treatment strategies and complications of appendicitis occuring during pregnancy

Chapter 4 - Fetal development is entirely dependent on the mother during pregnancy. Epidemiologic and clinical data suggest that immunologic and metabolic profiles of the pregnant uterus are responsive to mother's diet. This evidence supports the hypothesis that maternal nutrition may influence fetal programming and disease risk in the offspring. After birth, the gastrointestinal tract undergoes vast structural and functional adaptations under the stimulation of the microbiota and the diet that make possible handle with antigens and digest milk and latter solid food. The intestinal colonization process implies the activation of diverse metabolic functions either triggered by host-microbe interactions or directly encoded by the genome of the microbiota (microbiome). Moreover, microbial exposure through colonization process of the newborn intestine is essential to regulate epithelial permeability and immune function, with long-term consequences on host's health. Bacterial composition and succession during the intestinal colonization process have been shown to determine susceptibility to infections and sensitization to dietary antigens. In this context, mammals seem to have a developmental window within the perinatal and postnatal period, in which the host-gut microbiota interactions are more influential in favoring later health. Probiotic and prebiotic administration has been demonstrated to be a dietary strategy that at least temporary modulates the microbiota composition and may favor a healthy status. These strategies have demonstrated moderate efficacy to reduce the risk of infections and allergic diseases early in life. In recent years, the administration of probiotics to pregnant and lactating mothers in addition to their newborns, together or not with prebiotics, has also been evaluated to extend their applications and improve effectiveness by acting in these critical developmental stages. In this type of intervention, specific probiotic strains have been demonstrated to influence gut growth and immune function in the offspring of animal models. Other studies have suggested that this dietary strategy may help to reduce the risk of atopy, infections, and metabolic disorders in humans. The current knowledge on the effectiveness and mechanisms by which the administration of probiotics to mothers and infants can positively affect early stages of development, favoring latter heath are review.

Chapter 5 - *Background:* The gap between scientific knowledge and clinical practice is a major challenge in neonatal pain management. The aim of this study was to describe the clinicians' perceptions concerning the treatment of procedural pain in neonates, before and after the implementation of new pain-management strategies.

Methods: A multifaceted approach to changing practice was evaluated among nurses and physicians in two 16 beds neonatal intensive care units in southern Norway. The intervention included the establishment of an organizational framework for the change process, the development and implementation of evidence-based guidelines and procedures, education and local facilitators that assisted clinicians in changing their practice. Data were collected before and after the intervention, using a questionnaire. Ten commonly performed procedures were assessed. The response rates were 79% and 73%, respectively.

Results: Clinicians' answers indicated a slight increase in the actual use of pharmacological agents. Only the nurses reported changes in their views of procedure painfulness, the actual use of comfort measures, and the perceived optimal treatment for procedural pain. The intervention did not result in more concordant perceptions of physicians and nurses, neither in comprehensive changes in the treatment of procedural pain in neonates. Despite the performance of a multifaceted intervention to support evidence-based practice, the overall results point clearly to the difficulties in applying evidence to practice.

Chapter 6 - Data for the present work were based on electronic search of research studies published on the subject. The literature suggests that chances of malnutrition in infants considerably increase during natural disasters and crisis situations. In such emergencies, helping mothers successfully initiate and continue breastfeeding becomes even more crucial.

Children in vulnerable situations have special needs for infection-fighting factors, optimal nutrition, reliable food source and comfort; all these can be ensured only by breastfeeding. Usually the water sources are contaminated during emergencies and if used for dilution of powdered milk and/or washing of nipples and bottles, this water can cause irreversible health damage to the infants.

In contrast, human milk provides ample hydration and spares infants exposure to contaminated water due to destruction in emergencies. As rate of infections increases during emergencies; infants who are not breastfed will be more susceptible to infections and other illnesses. Consequently, they will be more likely to require hospitalization and to die in the first year of life, in fact, considerably costing the families and community. Mothers warrant extra support during crises; which demands for rapidly keeping their infants with them and providing space where they can feel comfortable nursing. Mothers delivering during the crisis should be encouraged and helped to initiate breastfeeding immediately after birth and to exclusive breastfeed for approximately 6 months.

Those mothers who recently stopped breastfeeding due to stress should be assisted to relactate. Misconceptions and fears leading to stop and/or minimize breastfeeding must be dispelled with accurate information. Wherever and whenever needed suitable arrangements for wet nursing must be made ensuring optimal infant nutritional requirements. Beside, proper feeding the mother is the safest, most effective way to ensure adequate infant nutrition during emergencies.

Versions of these chapters were also published in *International Journal of Medical and Biological Frontiers,* Volume 16, Numbers 1-2, 5-12, edited by Tsisana Shartava, published by Nova Science Publishers, Inc. They were submitted for appropriate modifications in an effort to encourage wider dissemination of research.

In: Pregnancy and Infants
Editor: Tsisana Shartava

ISBN 978-1-61209-132-7
© 2011 Nova Science Publishers, Inc.

Chapter 1

MULTIPLE SCLEROSIS DURING PREGNANCY

Yára Dadalti Fragoso *

Department of Neurology, Medical Faculty UNIMES
Rua da Constituição 374, Santos SP, Brazil

INTRODUCTION

Multiple sclerosis (MS) is more prevalent in women of childbearing age, posing an extra challenge in the management of this chronic neurological disease. For several decades, women with MS were discouraged from having children, until knowledge accumulated after the work of Confravreux et al [1] showed otherwise. In fact, current knowledge shows that the gestational period has a beneficial role in MS relapse rate without affecting the long-term progress of the disease [2]. Additionally, the recent therapeutic advances may help MS women to remain active for a long period of time, providing proper maternal care [3]. However, the relative lack of data from different countries and institutions, as well as the poor information on exposure to MS drugs, create the need for further research on the subject. It is unlikely that any trial

* E-mail: yara@bsnet.com.br

on current approved MS drugs will ever consider including pregnant women in the study. Therefore, this chapter summarizes literature data on the MS and pregnancy, discussing the effects of one condition onto the other, and reproductive risks for both mother and child. Many subsections of this chapter are based upon general concepts and several authors' personal opinions, since no evidence-based is available for some questions. Some symptoms of MS may determine different approaches to particular problems, without any evidence-based data. For example, spasticity of lower limbs may affect normal delivery and require cesarean intervention, as discussed forthwith. Other relevant issues of MS symptoms in pregnancy are also discussed along the chapter.

REPRODUCTIVE COUNSELING

As a general concept, women who suffer from potentially serious illnesses are considered to be of higher risk for pregnancy and its outcomes. Counseling on pregnancy in MS patients should include several professionals and the closest relative. The uncertainty of being able to care for a child due to the progressive physical and cognitive disability, as well as fatigue, is an important issue to be addressed. Obviously, the more aggressive the disease is, the higher the risks of not being able to provide adequate maternal care. It is also important to consider that more aggressive MS is usually treated with medications of higher fetal risk. Adequate pregnancy planning must consider interruption of immunomodulatory and/or immunosuppressive treatments for at least three months prior to conception. Therefore, only women with relative well-controlled disease activity should be encouraged to get pregnant.

COUNSELING ON GENETIC ISSUES

MS patients considering motherhood may be concerned on the genetic risks of the disease on their offspring. There is a polygenic pattern of transmission for MS, increasing the absolute risk of the disease to 2% to 4% [4]. Varying degrees of association with MS were described for class II DR2 halotypes of the human leukocyte antigen (HLA) DRB1*1501, DQB1*0602 and DQA1*0102, located on chromosome 6p21 [5, 6]. This association is observed in all ethnic groups, but it is particularly noticeable in Caucasians.

Recent studies in two independent European populations have shown higher susceptibility to MS associated with two single nucleotide polymorphisms (SNP) in genes IL2RA (rs12722489 and rs2104286), and with one SNP in the IL7RA gene (rs6897932) [7].

The evidence for increased MS risk in relatives of a patient should not be a deterrent for childbearing. Epidemiological studies and genomic screening suggest that the genetic influence on MS susceptibility is present, but relatively small and still controversial in several aspects [8, 9].

HORMONE-RELATED CHANGES IN PREGNANCY AND MS

Immunocompetent cells have hormone receptors in their surface, at least partially responsible for gender-related differences in neuroimmunological diseases [10]. The hormonal changes that occur in pregnancy induce a physiological shift from Th1 to Th2 immune response, yielding a favorable profile of anti-inflammatory cytokines (IL-4, IL-10, TGF-β) [10, 11]. This shift may be part of the reasons for the observed reduced relapse rate during pregnancy [1]. In addition, the decrease in CD56 (dim) natural killer cells (NK) during the third semester of the gestational period could also account for the significant reduction of relapses in this period [1, 12]. No changes on percentages of peripheral blood CD3, CD4, CD8 and CD19 immune cell subsets have been reported during the same period [12].

It was recently reported that estrogen induced the expression of indoleamine 2,3-dioxygenase (IDO) on monocyte-derived dendritic cells (DCs), limiting T-cell proliferation and both Th1 and Th2 cytokine production [13, 14]. The suppression of T-cell proliferation mediated by estrogen-exposed DCs was partly abolished by the IDO-inhibitor, 1-methyl-dl-tryptophan, indicating that estrogen-exposed DCs were capable of inducing IDO-dependent T-cell suppression [13].

The fetal-placental unit produces estriol, a type of estrogen that is probably responsible for part of the relative immunosuppressive state of pregnancy, since the fetus is an allograft carrying a variety of potential antigens. Estrogens, such as estriol, have been used in clinical trials outside pregnancy periods, and so far the results are still controversial [15-18].

Another substance typical of pregnancy is the alpha-fetoprotein, an oncofetal glycoprotein found in fetal and maternal fluids during pregnancy.

The suppressive effect of alpha-fetoprotein on T cells has been described over 30 years ago [19, 20], although no changes in the total number of these cells could be observed [21]. More recent animal studies have shown that T cells from treated mice had significantly reduced activity towards the encephalitogenic peptide of myelin oligodendrocyte glycoprotein (MOG) [22]. Alpha-fetoprotein also inhibited the MOG-specific antibody production and the expression of CD11b, MHC class II and the chemokine receptor CCR5 [22]. Recombinant human alpha-fetoprotein is now being considered as possible tool for autoimmune diseases [23], since the cytokines profile is potentially and beneficially altered [24]. The initial trials on the clinical use of alpha-fetoprotein for MS treatment showed that this protein is well tolerated, capable of decreasing various aspects of neuroinflammation, including disease severity, axonal loss and damage, T-cell reactivity, and antigen presentation [25].

In summary, all the maternal alterations induced by pregnancy have a positive effect on MS activity control. These beneficial changes are clinically reflected by the reduced relapse rate during the gestational period, a statement that no research is, as yet, opposed to.

FERTILITY AND CONCEPTION IN MS

There are no reports on specific physiological effects of MS on fertility and conception [3]. However, the high rates of sexual dysfunction reported in these patients [26] may be associated to a variety of neurological disabilities, affecting the overall quality of sexual life [27]. Weakness, spasticity, incoordenation, spasms, depression, bladder and bowel dysfunction, sleep disorders, pain, paroxysmal disorders and sensorial alterations may be serious deterrents for conception [28]. It is important to consider that many drugs used to treat these disabling conditions are not safe for use during pregnancy. In summary [29], the Food and Drug Administration (FDA) classification for drugs specifies that there are no safe, Class A, drugs. Class B includes drugs with no evidence of harm to the fetus, this being a conclusion achieved without a proper controlled trial. Class C includes drugs that deserve a special consideration on risk-benefit, since animal studies have shown a degree of harm to the fetus. Class D drugs with evidence of fetal risk, should only be considered in life-threatening situations or when safer drugs have proven to be inefficient. Drugs of extreme high risk, positively associated to birth defects, are considered to be class X and should not be used in potentially fertile women. Oxybutine used for incontinence and pemoline used for fatigue are Class B drugs according to the FDA classification. A variety of commonly used drugs for MS symptoms are classified as C drugs: baclofen and dantrolene for spasticity, gabapentin and carbamazepin for paroxysmal disorders and pain, amantadine and potassium channel blockers for fatigue, as well as the selective serotonin reuptake inhibitors frequently used for depression. Benzodiazepines and phenytoin used for pain and sleep disorders are Class D drugs.

The previously reported lower fertility in MS women [30] may be a reflection of a reduced propensity to maternity, particularly in cases with no proper counseling. Nevertheless, other factors may apply, such as the protracted or irreversible amenorrhea associated to the use of mitoxantrone [31].

MS TREATMENT DURING PREGNANCY

Immunomodulatory and immunosuppressive drugs used for MS treatment aim to reduce the frequency and severity of relapses, as well as to delay disability. According to the FDA classification, there are no safe, Class A, drugs. Class B drugs include immunoglobulin and glatiramer acetate. Class C includes beta-interferons, mitroxantrone and corticosteroids. Class D drugs include azathioprine and cyclophosphamide. Metothrexate is considered to be of very high risk of fetal malformation (Class X). Ideally, women intending to become pregnant should interrupt their treatment for at least three months prior to conception.

The literature on the subject reports only on a small number of pregnancies, not allowing firm conclusions to be drawn with regards to their safety of these drugs [32].

Specific studies on the subject (those including a special database designed for this purpose) in the last five years, report on populations from Sweden [33], Canada [34], Spain [35], Finland [36], Italy [37], and Germany [38]. The Swedish study, discussing effects of interferon beta 1a, concluded that pregnancies not exposed to the drug *in utero* for at least two weeks before conception resulted in more healthy infants than those exposed. Despite the small population on this study and the lack of statistically significant findings, this report concludes that it is advisable to stop interferon beta 1a before conception [33]. The Canadian study confirmed this conclusion, reporting on a small number of pregnancies exposed to interferon beta with significantly higher risks of abortion, low birth weight and prematurity [34].

The Spanish study included a higher number of patients and did not find a significantly higher rate of complications for those accidentally exposed to immunomodulators [35]. The Finnish group did not concentrate on drug exposure and its possible complications [36], while the Italian group concluded that there is no indication for pregnancy interruption in MS women exposed to interferon beta in the early stages of pregnancy [37].

The German study reported on higher incidence of low birth weight in mothers with MS, even without the use of immunomodulators [38]. Data on pregnancy complications from the recently licensed natalizumab are few, but a surveillance post-marketing program showed that all induced abortions performed in fear of birth malformations presented normal fetuses [29].

Due to the lack of definite data on the subject, it is generally recommended that women who intend to get pregnant should not be in use of medications of any kind. At the same time, women who could potentially become pregnant should preferentially receive Class B medications for MS and its symptoms, since there are no Class A drugs for these conditions according to the FDA.

MS AND DELIVERY

In general, the way of delivery is decided taking into consideration the obstetric indications rather than the presence of this neurological condition [3]. It is possible that lower limbs spasticity may become an indication for a cesarean section, but overall, the rates of cesarean operations is similar to those for women without MS [39]. Special attention should be given to pre-operative evaluation, in order to decrease neurological-related post-operative complications in these patients. Regarding the type of anesthesia, epidural injection seems to be safer than spinal block [40], since the latter has been previously reported to possibly be associated with a neurotoxic effect [41, 42]. General anesthesia, considered to be of high risk for MS patients, has proven to be safe in this population [42, 43]. Patients should be informed on the plan for anesthesia and be aware of possible complications.

Although very rare, and basically related to lesions on the spinal cord, autonomic dysreflexia can occur in MS patients [44]. In this condition, hypertension and compensatory parasympathetic overactivy may lead to complications [3], requiring vigorous intervention.

Data on the large Norwegian Medical Birth Registration showed that, independently of MS treatment and disease stage, the neonates were of lower birth weight and height, and more interventional delivery was reported [45-47].

RELAPSE RISK AFTER DELIVERY

The increased relapse risk after delivery, in comparison to the gestational period, is not contested by any research. In fact, the above discussed beneficial effects of pregnancy on MS course explain very well the changes noticed by all authors [3]. The risk for a relapse in the postpartum period is increased for women with higher relapse rates and higher EDSS before pregnancy [48]. The slightly longer hospitalization period for Ms mothers did not seem to relate to higher rates of complications, but rather to a more prudent attitude from the obstetricians [32].

Few studies discuss the rationale for using corticosteroids or immunoglobulin in the immediate postpartum period in order to avoid relapses in this period [49-52]. The data so far reported is encouraging, suggesting that such approach may indeed prevent higher relapse rates.

BREASTFEEDING

The higher risk for relapses in the postpartum period may lead the physicians to discourage breastfeeding, in order to resume immunomodulatory or immunosuppressive treatment in these patients. However, due to the scarce data on the subject, most decisions are taken individually, without evidence-based studies. An American survey showed that only 11% of all physicians allow medications in the breastfeeding period, mostly glatiramer acetate [53].

The same survey showed that neurologists preferred to leave the decision on breastfeeding to the patient. The transfer of large molecules, such as interferon beta, to the human milk is unlikely to be significant.

There are no studies regarding the levels of immunomodulatory and immunosuppressive MS drugs on the human milk and, indeed, if the oral intake of these amounts by the child could be significant. As a general rule,

breastfeeding can be allowed in women using FDA Class A or B drugs –
although for Class B, breastfeeding could be intercalated with bottled milk
formulas, reducing the risk of excessive exposure.

LONG-TERM EFFECTS OF PREGNANCY ON MS

The long-term relapse rate and disease evolution do not seem to be
affected by pregnancy in MS patients. There are no reports to that effect, and
major reviews emphasize that, on the long term, pregnancy does not alter MS
course [2, 3, 29, 36].

CONCLUSION

Women with MS must be reassured that pregnancy, in itself, does not
seem to negatively affect the disease and that MS does not negatively affect
pregnancy outcomes. The decision on motherhood has been studied and
reported recently [54]. Women seemed to be mainly concerned with their own
health and well-being, the well-being of the child, the difficulties in
experiencing and coping with parenthood, with social attitudes and also the
pressure on decision making [54].

The obvious lack of double-blind, controlled data on drugs prior, during,
and immediately after pregnancy has created the need for databases on drug
exposure. There are only a few studies addressing this issue. The importance
of the subject *MS and pregnancy* requires further collaborative, international
studies on the matter before firmer conclusions can be obtained. Lack of
knowledge has lead to several induced abortions of normal fetuses and still
creates a high degree of anxiety and insecurity among women with MS and
their relatives, as well as among obstetricians and neurologists caring for these
patients.

REFERENCES

[1]   Confravreux C; Hutchinson M; Hours MM; Cortinovis-Tourniaire P;
       Moreau T. Rate of pregnancy-related relapse in multiple sclerosis. *N.
       Eng J. Med.*; 1998;339:283–291.

[2] Bennett KA. Pregnancy and multiple sclerosis. *Clin. Obstet Gynecol.* 2005;48:38-47.

[3] Argyriou AA and Makris N. Multiple sclerosis and reproductive risks in women. *Reprod. Sci.* 2008;15:755-64.

[4] Dyment DA; Ebers GC; Sadovnick AD. Genetics of multiple sclerosis. *Lancet Neurol* 2004;3:104-10.

[5] Kantarci O and Wingerchuk D. Epidemiology and natural risk of multiple sclerosis: new insights. *Curr. Opin. Neurol.* 2006;19:248-54.

[6] Ramagopalan SV; McMahon R; Dyment DA; Sadovinik AD; Ebers GC; Wittkowski KM. An extension to a statistical approach for family based association studies provides insights into genetic risk factors for multiple sclerosis in the HLA-DRB1 gene. *BMC Med. Genet.* 2009;10:10.

[7] Weber F; Fontaine B; Cournu-Rebeix I; Kroner A; Knop M; Lutz S; Müller-Sarnowisk F; Uhr M; Bettecken T; Kohli M; Ripke S; Ising M; Rieckmann P; Brassat D; Semana G; Babron MC; Mrejen S; Gout C; Lyon-Caen O; Yaouang J; Edan G; Clanet M; Holsboer F; Clerget-Darpoux F; Müller-Myhsok B. IL2RA and IL7RA genes confer susceptibility for multiple sclerosis in two independent European populations. *Genes Immun.* 2008;9:259-63.

[8] Oksenberg JR and Barcellos LF. The complex genetic aetiology of multiple sclerosis. *J. Neurovirol.* 2000;6(suppl 2):S10-S14.

[9] Schmidt H; Williamson D; Ashley-Koch A. HLA-DR15 haplotype and multiple sclerosis: a HuGE review. *Am. J. Epidemiol.* 2007; 165:1097:109.

[10] Devonshire V; Duquette P; Dwosh E; Guimond C; Sadovinik AD. The immune system and hormones: review and relevance to pregnancy and contraception in women with MS. *Int. MS. J.* 2003;10:61-6.

[11] Robertson SA; Seamark RF; Gilbert LJ; Wegmann TG. The role of cytokines in gestation. *Crit. Rev. Immunol.* 1994;14:239-92.

[12] Airas L; Saraste M; Rinta S; Elovaara I; Huang YH; Wiendl H; Finnish multiple sclerosis and pregnancy study group. Immunoregulatory factors in multiple sclerosis patients during and after pregnancy: relevance of natural killer cells. *Clin. Exp. Immunol.* 2008;151:235-43.

[13] Zhu WH; Lu CZ;huang YM; Link H; Xiao BG. A putative mechanism on remission of multiple sclerosis during pregnancy: estrogen-induced indoleamine 2;3-dioxygenase by dendritic cells. *Mult. Scler.* 2007;13:33-40.

[14] Kahler DJ and Mellor AR. T cell regulatory plasmacytoid dendritic cells expressing indoleamine 2;3 dioxygenase. *Handb Exp. Pharmacol.* 2009; 188:165-96.

[15] Antonio M; Patrizia F; Ilaria I; Paolo F. A rational approach on the use of sex steroids in multiple sclerosis. *Recent Pat CNS Drug. Discov.* 2008;3:34-9.

[16] Tanzer J. Estrogen effect in multiple sclerosis more nuanced than described. *Ann. Neurol.* 2008;63:263.

[17] Salem ML. Estrogen; a double-edged sword: modulation of TH1- and TH2-mediated inflammations by differential regulation of TH1/TH2 cytokine production. *Curr. Drug Targets Inflamm Allergy* 2004;3:97-104.

[18] Soldan SS; Alvarez Retuerto AI; Sicotte NL; Voskhul RR. Immune modulation in multiple sclerosis patients treated with the pregnancy hormone estriol. *J. Immunol.* 2003;171:6267-74.

[19] Murgita RA; Andersson LC; Sherman MS; Bennich H; Wigzell H. Effects of human alpha-fetoprotein on human B and T lymphocyte proliferation *in vitro*. Clin Exp Immunol; 1978;33: 347–56.

[20] Stahn R. Suppression of human T-cell colony formation during pregnancy. *Nature* 1978;276:831-2.

[21] Birk K; Ford C; Smeltzer S; Ryan D; Miller R; Rudick RA. Clinical course of Multiple Sclerosis during pregnancy and the puerperium. *Arch. Neurol.* 1990;47:738-42.

[22] Irony-Tur-Sinai M; Gligoriadis N; Lourbopoulos A; Pinto-Maaravi F; Abramsky O; Brenner I. Amelioration of autoimmune neuro-inflammation by recombinant human alpha-fetoprotein. *Exp. Neurol.* 2006;198:136-44.

[23] Dudich E. MM-093, a recombinant human alpha-fetoprotein for the potential treatment of rheumatoid arthritis and other autoimmune diseases. *Curr. Opin. Mol. Ther* 2007;9:603-10.

[24] McClain MA; Gatson NN; Powell ND; Papenfuss TL; Gienapp IE; Song F; Shawler TM; Kithcart A; Whitacre CC. Pregnancy suppresses experimental autoimmune encephalomyelitis through immunoregulatory cytokine production. *J. Immunol.* 2007;15:8146-52.

[25] Nizri E; Irony-Tur-Sinai M; Grigoriadis N; Abramsky O; Amitai G; Brenner T. Novel approaches to treatment of autoimmune neuroinflammation and lessons for drug development. *Pharmacol.* 2007;79:42-9.

[26] Fletcher SG; Castro-Borrero W; Remington G; Treadaway K; Lemack GE; Frohman EM. Sexual dysfunction in patients with multiple sclerosis: a multidisciplinary approach to evaluation and management. *Nat. Clin. Pract Urol.* 2009;6:96-107.

[27] Tepavcevic DK; Kostic J; Basuroski ID; Stojsavljevic N; Pekmezovic T; Drulovic J. The impact of sexual dysfunction on the quality of life measured by MSQoL-54 in patients with multiple sclerosis. *Mult. Scler.* 2008 Sep;14(8):1131-6.

[28] Demirkiran M; Sarica Y; Uguz S; Yerdelen D; Aslan K. Multiple sclerosis patients with and without sexual dysfunction: are there any differences? *Mult. Scler.* 2006;12:209-14.

[29] Ghezzi A and Zaffaroni M. Female-specific issues in multiple sclerosis. *Exp. Ver. Neurotherapeutics* 2008;8:969-77.

[30] Runmarker B and Andersen O. Pregnancy is associated with a lower risk of onset and a better prognosis in multiple sclerosis. *Brain* 1995;118:253–61.

[31] Cocco E; Sardu C; Gallo P; Capra R; Amato MP; Trojano M; Uccelli A; Marrosu MG; FEMIMS group. Frequency and risk factors of mitoxantrone-induced amenorrhea in multiple sclerosis: the FEMIMS study. *Mult. Scler* 2008;14:1225-33.

[32] Ferrero S; Esposito F; Pretta S; Ragni N. Fetal risks related to the treatment of multiple sclerosis during pregnancy and breastfeeding. *Exp. Rev. Neurother* 2006;6:1823-31.

[33] Sandberg-Wollheim M; Frank D; Goodwin TM; Giesser B; Lopez-Bresnahan M; Stam-Moraga M; Chang P; Francis GS. Pregnancy outcomes during treatment with interferon beta-1a in patients with multiple sclerosis. *Neurology* 2005;65:802-6.

[34] Boskovic R; Wide R; Wolpin J; Bauer DJ; koren G. The reproductive effects of beta interferon therapy in pregnancy: a longitudinal cohort. *Neurology* 2005;65:807-11.

[35] De las Heras V; De Andres C; Tellez N; Tintore M. Pregnancy in multiple sclerosis patients treated with immunomodulators prior to or during part of the pregnancy: a descriptive study in the Spanish population. *Mult Scler* 2007;13:981-4.

[36] Saraste M; Väisänen S; Alanen A; Airas L; Finnish Multiple Sclerosis And Pregnancy Study Group. Clinical and immunologic evaluation of women with multiple sclerosis during and after pregnancy. *Gend Med.* 2007;4:45-55.

[37] Patti F; Cavallaro T; Lo Fermo S; Nicoletti A; Cimino V; Vecchio R; Laisa P; Zarbo R; Zappia M. Is in utero early-exposure to interferon beta a risk factor for pregnancy outcomes in multiple sclerosis? *J. Neurol.* 2008;255:1250-3.

[38] Hellwig K; Brune N; Haghikia A; Muller T; Schimrigk S; Schwodiauer V; Gold R. Reproductive counseling; treatment and course of pregnancy in 73 German MS patients. *Acta Neurol. Scand*; 2008;118:24-8.

[39] Mueller BA; Zhang J; Critchlow CW. Birth outcomes and need for hospitalization after delivery among women with multiple sclerosis. *Am. J. Obstet Gynecol.* 2002; 186:446-52.

[40] Dorotta IR and Schubert A. Multiple sclerosis and anesthetic implycations. *Curr. Opin. Anaesthesiol* 2002;15:365-70.

[41] Capdeville M and Hoyt MR. Anesthesia and analgesia in the obstetric population with multiple sclerosis. A retrospective review. *Anesthesiology* 1994; 81:1173.

[42] Vercauteren M and Heytens L. Anesthetic considerations for patients with a pre-existing neurological deficit: are neuraxial techniques safe? *Acta anaesthesiol Scand* 2007;51:831-8.

[43] Drake E; Drake M; Bird J; Russell R. Obstetric regional blocks for women with multiple sclerosis: a survey of the UK experience. *Int. J. Obstet Anesth.* 2006;15:115-23.

[44] Bateman AM and Goldish GD. Autonomic dysreflexia in multiple sclerosis. *J. Spinal. Cord. Med.* 2002;25:40-2.

[45] Dahl J; Myhr KM; Daltveit AK; Hoff JM; Gilhus NE. Pregnancy, delivery and birth outcome in women with multiple sclerosis. *Neurology* 2005;65:1961-3.

[46] Dahl J; Myhr KM; Daltveit AK; Gilhus NE. Planned vaginal births in women with multiple sclerosis. Delivery and birth outcomes. *Acta Neurol. Scand.* 2006;183:51-4.

[47] Dahl J; Myhr KM; Daltveit AK; Gilhus NE. Pregnancy, delivery and birth outcome in different stages of maternal multiple sclerosis. *J. Neurol.* 2008;255:623-7.

[48] Vukusic S; Hutchinson M; Hours M; Moreau T; Cortinovis- Tourniaire P; Adeleine P; Confavreux C; The Pregnancy In Multiple Sclerosis Group. *Brain* 2004;127:1353-60.

[49] De Seze J; Chapelotte M; Delalande S; Ferriby D; Stojkovic T; Vermersch P. Intravenous corticosteroids in the postpartum period for reduction of acute exacerbations in multiple sclerosis; *Mult Scler* 2004;10:596-7.

[50] Achiron A; Kishner I; Dolev M; Stern Y; Dulitzky M; Schiff E; Achiron R. Effect of intravenous immunoglobulin treatment on pregnancy and postpartum-related relapses in multiple sclerosis. *J. Neurol.* 2004; 251:1133-7.

[51] Ringel I and Zettl UK. Intravenous immunoglobulin therapy in neurological diseases during pregnancy. *J. Neurol.* 2006; 253[suppl 5]:V70-V74.

[52] Hellwig K; Beste C; Schimrigk S; Chan A. Immunomodulation and postpartum relapses in patients with multiple sclerosis. *Ther Adv. Neurol. Disorders* 2009;1:7-11.

[53] Coyle PK; Christie S; Fodor P; Fuchs K; Giesser B; Gutierrez A; Lynn J; Weinstock-Guttman B; Pardo L; Women Neurologists MS Initiative. Multiple sclerosis gender issues: clinical practices of women neurologists. *Mult. Scler.* 2004;10:582-8.

[54] Houtchens MK. Pregnancy and multiple sclerosis. *Semin. Neurol.* 2007;27:434-41.

In: Pregnancy and Infants   ISBN 978-1-61209-132-7
Editor: Tsisana Shartava   © 2011 Nova Science Publishers, Inc.

Chapter 2

PREGNANCY OUTCOME OF PATIENTS WITH CELIAC DISEASE

*Rachel Pope and Eyal Sheiner**

Departments of Obstetrics and Gynecology,
Soroka University Medical Center, and Faculty of Health Sciences,
Ben-Gurion University of the Negev, Beer-Sheva, Israel

ABSTRACT

Celiac disease, i.e. permanent intolerance to gluten, has an autoimmune mechanism. Controversy exists in the literature regarding the association between celiac and infertility, abortions, intra-uterine growth restriction (IUGR) and stillbirths. When properly managed, celiac disease might have little effect on pregnancy and birth outcomes. However, as a commonly undiagnosed disease, fertility, pregnancy, and birth might all be negatively affected by it when it is unrecognized and untreated. When celiac disease is untreated, women may be subfertile, or suffer infertility. If a woman manages to become pregnant without

* Corresponding author: Eyal Sheiner, M.D, PhD., Department of Obstetrics and Gynecology, Soroka University Medical Center, P.O Box 151, Beer-Sheva, Israel. Tel 972-8-6403551 Fax 972-8-6403294. E-mail: sheiner@bgu.ac.il

treating celiac disease, there are higher rates of IUGR, and low birthweight (LBW) of her offspring. Therefore, celiac disease should be considered among idiopathic infertility repeat spontaneous abortion, and immediately and strictly treated in order to correct future risks. Control of a gluten-free diet is important in terms of healthy reproduction. Further, studies should focus on screening for celiac disease among patients presenting with IUGR of an unknown etiology.

Keywords: Pregnancy, Celiac Disease, Intrauterine growth restriction, Fertility.

I. INTRODUCTION

Permanent intolerance to gluten, known as celiac disease, affects both female and male fertility and pregnancy outcomes when untreated. Research suggests that infertility is correctable through treatment [1,2]; however, contradicting research results demonstrate discrepancies in pregnancy outcome possibly based on diagnosis and treatment. For example, just as in undiagnosed celiac women, higher rates of gestational disturbances leading to intrauterine growth restriction (IUGR,) low birth weight (LBW), and preterm delivery have also been found among diagnosed and presumably treated celiac men and women. [3,4,5,6] Moreover, several studies suggest that adverse effects of undiagnosed celiac disease are improved by treatment, [1,7] while other research has not been able to demonstrate any significant differences in pregnancy outcome from the rest of the population even when undiagnosed. [8,9] This may be do to screening discrepancies.

Celiac disease is estimated to affect anywhere from 1 in 85 to 300 persons in populations of European decent; however it has been reported among other populations who have immigrated to western countries. [10] Besides particular populations, celiac disease also tends to affect certain individuals more than others. For example, individuals with other autoimmune immune diseases such as Crohn's disease or lupus often have celiac disease as an autoimmune comorbidity. [11] Celiac disease is found in 2-5% of individuals with insulin-dependent diabetes mellitus or autoimmune thyroid disease. [11] In addition, celiac disease has been found to be significantly under-diagnosed, but most closely linked to anemia of varying severity and therefore should also be considered for these patients. [12] Regardless of risk factors, individuals need to be aware of disease status and how to manage celiac disease. Therefore, screening should be considered for women and men experiencing idiopathic infertility as well as men and women at particular risk because of population or other autoimmune diseases.

Although exact etiology of celiac disease remains unknown, several postulations have been made and investigated in relation to its effects on reproduction. For example, reproductive disorders could be due to nutritional defects instigated by celiac disease [13] However, no studies have yet been able to demonstrate this. One study that investigated folic acid deficiency as a possible side effect of celiac disease showed that the deficiency was due to metabolism and not absorption, and therefore, not necessarily associated with celiac disease [14]. Other experts suggest that the high number of autoantibodies acting against self-antigens could indicate self antibodies against hormones and organs necessary for normal pubertal and hormonal development, or selective malabsorption of micronutrients needed for metabolism of carrier or receptor proteins for sex hormones [15] Treatment entails a life-long elimination of gluten from the diet.

A literature review conducted by Eliakim and Sherer of the information linking celiac disease and pregnancy from 1966 to 2000 revealed that patients with untreated celiac disease sustain a significantly delayed menarche, earlier menopause, and an increased prevalence of secondary amenorrhea [1] They went on to explain that patients with untreated celiac disease incur higher miscarriage rates, increased fetal growth restriction, and lower birth weights and that improvement of celiac disease, as reflected by restoration of small bowel mucosa associated with implementation of a gluten-free diet, may decrease miscarriage rates, improve fetal nutritional support and overall perinatal outcome. However, more recent research shows that such improvements may not be dependent upon treatment.

II. CELIAC AND FERTILITY

Deeper investigations into idiopathic infertility reveal a higher prevalence of celiac disease than the average population, estimated at 4-8% of women with unexplained infertility as compared to 0.3-1.2%. [16,17,18] However, when treated, fertility may be attained at normal population rates giving evidence that celiac disease is a major deterrent of fertility when untreated [18] Therefore, these affected individuals wishing to conceive should also receive screening and counseling for celiac disease. North American and Western Europeans have a higher rate of celiac disease than the rest of the world's population and therefore, screening should be considered if experiencing fertility problems. Because celiac disease is well-established as a genetic disease, individuals with a first-degree relative with celiac disease and are wishing to conceive might also be screened [19]

A. Shorter Reproductive Period

In general, women with celiac disease have a shorter reproductive window than the average population. Literature indicates that women with untreated celiac disease experience menarche at a significantly later age when compared to the general population [20] Besides the typical signs and symptoms affecting the gastrointestinal tract, celiac disease may also present as hypogonadism which leads to the delayed menstrual cycle when untreated [15] Onset of menarche may be regulated, however, by a gluten-free diet [20].

Females affected by celiac disease also tend to have an increased prevalence of secondary amenorrhea, earlier onset of menopause, and fewer children [20] Any one of these disruptions in ovulation results in a shortened window of reproductive period and therefore results in less opportunity for fertility. However, a late onset menarche is not specific enough to indicate celiac disease, and therefore, many women with celiac disease are unaware of their status. In these cases, subfertility may be the first symptom of celiac disease [11] Since celiac disease presents with various symptoms and at various stages of life; onset may not occur until adulthood and even then, symptoms may be nonspecific or "silent." [16] Though subfertility is not the most common presentation of celiac disease in a person suffering from celiac disease, it is entirely possibly that women who are having trouble conceiving are affected significantly from this silent disease. Because the mechanism is not yet known, it is also unclear whether the nature of the silent form of the disease also prevents women from conceiving or if it those that have obvious symptoms are more likely to treat their disease and therefore escape fertility problems. Therefore, a study to examine the fertility of women with known celiac disease compared to the general population helps to clarify this discrepancy. Such a study found that women with known celiac disease experience similar fertility and birth outcomes compared to the general population [21]

The only distinction regarding fertility is the age at which the women conceived. Celiac women of younger reproductive age had lower fertility rates compared to controls, while older celiac women had higher fertility rates. However, the authors attributed this outcome of shifted fertility to the trend of socioeconomic and educational advantages of women with known celiac disease.

Therefore, the findings may have more to do with the fact that women who are aware of their disease have children later in life for reasons other than their disease status and in general, women with treated celiac disease can achieve fertility comparable to the general population. Regardless, women with diagnosed celiac disease can achieve improved fertility outcomes [20]

B. Male Infertility

Although less obvious than female adolescents, males with celiac disease present with a reduced serum level of dihydrotestosterone and an increased serum level of luteinizing hormone, suggesting androgen resistance [17] Elevated LH levels and free testosterone in men is a parallel hormone imbalance to polycystic ovarian syndrome (PCOS) in females, however a significant correlation between celiac and PCOS has not been demonstrated [22] Because of such hormone imbalances, celiac disease may also affect male fertility. When compared to other autoimmune diseases like Crohn's disease, celiac disease has a more significant impact on fertility and therefore has mechanics beyond malnutrition [23] Affected men have an exaggerated gonadotropin response to gonadotropin-releasing hormone implying an underlying pituitary problem; however, no studies have been done to demonstrate the effect of improved diet and control of celiac disease on male fertility since the 1970's. [2,23] Therefore, men also experiencing problems conceiving should be screened for celiac disease. However, it is not clear that treatment of the disease will improve all pregnancy outcomes as even treated celiac disease in either parent can lead to LBW and shorter duration of pregnancy, indicating a stronger case for genetic etiology [24]

III. CELIAC DURING PREGNANCY

Mixed results of celiac's effect on pregnancy deserve further examination. Two primary problems with research thus far has been that many are retrospective studies and lack clear definitions of severity of the disease as well as degree of management of the disease. Several studies have found that celiac women who do achieve fertilization, often have higher chances of miscarriages, IUGR, lower birth weight, still births, and shorter duration of breastfeeding [3,4] Like infertility, these gestational problems can also be the first symptom of celiac disease in an adult woman. IUGR is associated with vascular endometrium abnormalities and malfunction in implantation and trophoblastic endometrial invasion, though precise pathogenesis has not yet been solidified [25] Sheiner et al. found that there was no difference in pregnancy outcomes between celiac women and controls except that celiac women tend to also be anemic and IUGR persists as a gestational morbidity and therefore needs to be carefully followed and managed [5] Fetal IUGR conveys a significant risk of perinatal morbidity and mortality. When due to a maternal disease, the failure to achieve optimal weight can be due to a spectrum of factors including inadequate substrates for fetal metabolism and decreased oxygen availability or access. Therefore, fetal growth must be monitored with ultrasound throughout the pregnancy and elimination of gluten from the diet if celiac disease is suspected [26]

"Silent" or undiagnosed celiac disease is associated with recurrent spontaneous abortions. [7, 27] One study found that spontaneous abortion is more likely among women with untreated celiac disease than among the general population and women on a gluten free diet. [28] Similarly, the relative risk of abortion in untreated women was almost nine times higher than those treated according to Ciacci et al.'s study [29] Martinelli and Norgard have showed that improved outcomes are possible after one year of a gluten-free diet, highlighting the importance of diagnosis and treatment [7,4] Contrarily, Ferguson et al. showed that maternal health was not seriously impaired by pregnancy in patients with undiagnosed celiac in their study, although those on a gluten-free diet had significantly fewer symptoms and had heavier babies [27] Similarly, Kolho was not able to demonstrate significantly increased prevalence of celiac disease among women with recurrent miscarriage [9] Therefore, it is possible that the mothers with higher adverse effects on pregnancy are also those individuals with more severe cases of celiac disease [8] Improved screening techniques have found increasing numbers of silent forms of the disease among pregnant women and fewer adverse outcomes indicating that the rate of unfavorable events of pregnancy in celiac patients may not be significantly different from that observed in the non-celiac population [8]

Research results have shown that there are also adverse affects during pregnancy with males who have celiac disease, further indicating that genetics may have a strong effect on celiac disease and pregnancy outcome and that adverse pregnancy is not necessarily preventable through diagnosis and diet modification. Therefore, pregnancy of celiac women ought to be carefully monitored. Regardless of pregnancy prognoses, untreated celiac disease can in general cause anemia and discomfort and is therefore worth diagnosing and treating [5,12]

IV. SCREENING

Although complete diagnostic procedures including intestinal biopsy might be too dangerous for a pregnant woman, antiendomysial and antitissue transglutaminase antibody tests are specific and highly sensitive for celiac disease. The high positive predictive value of antibody testing can make the diagnosis almost certain, though generally, clinical or histological improvement while on a gluten-free diet should be demonstrated including a small intestinal biopsy to show the hallmark mucosal lesions that diagnose celiac disease.[13] Therefore, it is important that if warranted, screening occur before pregnancy in order to clarify the disease and in order to adequately manage it through dietary modifications.

V. TREATMENT

Infertility as presentation of celiac disease can give opportunity to initiate treatment for an otherwise asymptomatic disorder silently affecting a woman's health [13] Anecdotes of women with unexplained infertility, diagnosed with celiac disease, put on gluten-free diet, and successfully conceived have been documented [28,30] Just as symptoms of celiac disease in general can be resolved by a gluten-free diet, most reproductive problems can also be ameliorated in severe cases of celiac disease, although as previously explained, several authors have found that gestational diseases may still persist [5,6] Most of the studies conducted, however, have not had a very precise way of determining the adherence to a gluten-free diet and correlating it with birth outcome, therefore, there is ambiguity between diagnosed celiac disease and treated celiac disease. Furthermore, because of the nature of the retrospective studies, most that indicate a negative effect on pregnancy are of women with severe clinical presentation of celiac disease, and those showing little to no effect use methods of identification through a more sensitive screening that also diagnose "silent" cases. Hence, it is difficult to determine the actual pregnancy outcome when one manages the disease.

From the studies that screen women and men, it is evident that these individual's outcomes represent those who have not yet treated the disease through the course of the conception and pregnancy. These studies therefore, clearly show detrimental effects of both fertility and gestation [4] However, in retrospective studies of diagnosed celiac individuals, it is not clear how well the participants are managing the disease and therefore, outcomes from these studies are less reliable. Martinelli attempts to extract this discrepancy and shows that 7 out of 12 women who were diagnosed but not following a gluten-free diet had unfavorable outcomes in their pregnancies, while six women out of a total of 15 women with celiac disease, followed a gluten-free diet for one year and had healthy infants without problems [7] Norgard also showed that among the same women, once diagnosed with celiac disease, they had better birth outcomes than before, and assumed this is due to management of the disease [4] Unfortunately, conflicting evidence suggests that more powerful and precise research is needed.

Table 1. Incidence of Undiagnosed/untreated celiac women with idiopathic infertility

Women with idiopathic infertility that led to celiac diagnosis	Total number of idiopathic infertility	Percent and significance	Author
4	98	4.1% p=0.02	Collin 1996
4	99	4.0% P<0.03	Meloni 1999
1	47	2.0%	Kolho 1999

Table 2. Prevalence of unknown celiac disease among pregnant women

Percent unknown celiac disease	n	Type of study	Significantly unfavorable outcomes of those with celiac disease	Population	Author
1.4%	845	Hospital-based	58.3%	Campania, Italy	Martinelli 2000
1.3%	5055	Population based	0%	Campania, Italy	Greco 2004

Table 3.Number of women with celiac disease among those with miscarriage and IUGR

Percentage of celiac women with miscarriage or RSA	Percentage of celiac women with IUGR	Author
0%	--	Collin 1996
7.5%	15.4%	Gasbarrini 2000
5.8%	--	Sher 1996

Status of celiac disease	Type	n	Finding	Author	Year
Unknown	Cohort	5055	No excess risk of abortion, premature delivery, small birth weight, or IUGR. Anemia was more frequent in cases than controls.	Greco	2004
Unknown	Cohort	63	No association between celiac disease and recurrent abortion	Kolho	1999
Unknown	Cohort	845	The outcome of pregnancy was unfavorable in seven of 12 women with celiac disease. Six healthy babies were born with no problems after the women had been on a gluten free diet for one year.	Martinelli	2000
Unknown	Case-control	83 cases and 50 controls	The relative risk of IUGR and LBW could be 3-6 times higher than those with treated	Gasbarrini	2000

Table 3 (Continued)

Known	Retrospective	48	No difference with celiac women except for increased risks of IUGR and induction among women with celiac disease	Sheiner	2006
Known	Historical cohort	211 cases and 1260 controls	Celiac women had larger babies than control, women with unknown celiac had smaller babies and increased risk of IUGR; 3 times higher risk of IUGR with untreated disease	Norgard	1999
Known	Case-control	50	No higher prevalence of celiac disease among women with miscarriages compared to general population	Collin	1996
Known	Case-control	10597	whose father suffered from celiac disease had a lower birth weight (95% adjusted confidence interval (CI) — 459, —72 g), more often belonged to the low birth weight (LBW) category (LBW ≤2499 g) (95% CI adjusted odds ratio (AOR) 1.48-17.18), and had a shorter pregnancy duration (95% adjusted CI —1.53, —0.08 weeks) than non-celiac controls.	Ludvigsson and Ludvigsson	2001
Known	Case-control	80 cases and 70 controls	Appropriate treatment appears to eliminate risks. No higher incidences of infertility among women on gluten free diets	Sher	1996

CONCLUSION

Celiac disease causes subfertility and adverse pregnancy outcomes when untreated. Although infertility in either parent may be reversed through proper dietary management of the disease, adverse pregnancy outcomes are still possible. Although it is more likely that severe cases of celiac disease can be improved by dietary change, silent cases may unknowingly afflict gestation. Improvement in any manner through dietary management should be sought.

North Americans and Western Europeans are particularly at risk as well as individuals with another autoimmune disease, and/or a first-degree relative with celiac disease. If subfertile, these individuals may be screened for celiac disease. Patients may present as anemic and therefore, special attention needs to be given in these cases. Regardless of precise risk according to degree of disease severity, if any outcome may be improved by simply modifying the diet, women should be screened and made aware of their status. However, this should happen before she becomes pregnant since the intestinal biopsy of the complete diagnosis is risky while pregnant. If one is particularly concerned, an antibody test may be conducted and provide rather accurate results.

REFERENCES

[1]   Eliakim and Sherer Celiac disease: fertility and pregnancy. - *Gynecol Obstet Invest*, 2001; 51(1):3-7.

[2]   Baker Baker PG, Read AE. Reversible infertility in male coeliac patients. *BMJ* 1975;2:316–317.

[3]   Meloni GF, Dessole S, Vargiu N, Tomasi PA, and Musumeci S. The prevalence of coeliac disease in infertility. *Human Reproduction*, 1999.

[4]   Norgard B, Fonager K, Sorensen HT, Olsen J. Birth outcomes of women with celiac disease: a nationwide historical cohort study. *American Journal of Gastroenterology*. 1999:94;9:2435-2440.

[5]   Sheiner E, Peleg R, Levy A. Pregnancy outcome of patients with known celiac disease. *Eur. J. Obstet. Gynecol. Reprod. Biol.*, 2006:129(1):41-5.

[6]   Ludvigsson JF, Ludvigsson J. Coeliac disease in the father affects the newborn. *Gut* 2001;49:169–175.

[7]   Martinelli P, Troncone R, Paparo F, Torre P, Trapanese E, Fasano C, Lamberti A, Budillon G, Nardone G, Greco L. Coeliac disease and unfavourable outcome of pregnancy. *Gut*. 2000 Mar;46(3):332-5.

[8]   Greco L,Veneziano A, Di Donato L, Zampella C. Pecoraro M, Paladini D, Paparo F, Vollaro A, Martinelli P. Undiagnosed coeliac disease does not appear to be associated with unfavourable outcome of pregnancy. *Gut*. 2004 53:149-151.

[9]   Kolho K.-L., Tiitinen A, Tulppala M, Unkila-Kallio L, Savilahti. Screening for coeliac disease in women with a history of recurrent miscarriage or infertility - all 4 versions. BJOG: *An International Journal of Obstetrics and Gynaecology*, 1999; 106 (2) , 171–173.

[10] Lebenthal E, Branski D. Celiac disease: an emerging global problem. *J. Pediatr. Gastroenterol. Nutr.* 2002;35:472–474.

[11] Collin P, Kaukinen K, Valimaki M, et al. Endocrinological disorders and celiac disease. *Endocr. Rev.* 2002;23:464–483.

[12] Hin H, Bird G, Fisher P, et al. Coeliac disease in primary care: case finding study. *BMJ* 1999;318:164–167.

[13] Rostami K, Steegers EA, Wong WY, et al. Coeliac disease and reproductive disorders: a neglected association. *Eur. J. Obstet .Gynecol Reprod Biol.* 2001;96:146–149.

[14] Dickey W, Stewart F, Nelson J, et al. Screening for celiac disease as a possible maternal risk factor for neural tube defect. *Clin. Genet* 1996;49:107–108.

[15] Bona G, Marinello D, Oderda G, Mechanisms of Abnormal Puberty in Coeliac Disease. *Horm. Res.* 2002;57:63-65. 2002.

[16] Bradley RJ, Rosen MP. Subfertility and Gastrointestinal Disease: 'Unexplained'Is Often Undiagnosed. *Obstetrical and Gynecological Survey*, 2004. 59(2):108-117.

[17] Collin P, Vilska S, Heinonen PK, et al. Infertility and celiac disease. *Gut* 1996;39:382–384.

[18] Sher KS, Mayberry JF. Female fertility, obstetric and gynaecological history in coeliac disease: a case control study. *Acta Paediatr. Suppl.* 1996;412:76–77.

[19] Hogberg L, Falth-Magnusson K, Grodzinsky E, et al. Familial prevalence of coeliac disease: a twenty-year follow-up study. *Scand. J. Gastroenterol* 2003;38:61–65.

[20] Rujner J. Age at menarche in girls with celiac disease. Ginekol Pol 1999;70:359–362.

[21] Tata L , Card T , Logan R, Hubbard R, Smith C, West J. Fertility and pregnancy-related events in women with celiac disease: A population-based cohort study. *Gastroenterology.* 1999;128;4 :849 - 855

[22] Kuscu NK, Akcali S, Kucukmetin NT. Celiac disease and polycystic ovary syndrome. *Int. J. Gynaeco.*

[23] Farthing MJ, Rees LH, Edwards CR, et al. Male gonadal function in coeliac disease: 2. Sex hormones. *Gut* 1983;24: 127–135.

[24] Ludvigsson JF, Ludvigsson J. Coeliac disease in the father affects the newborn. *Gut* 2001;49:169–175.

[25] Daya, S. Eval and management of RAS *Curr. Opin. Obstet.Gyne* 1996: 8: 188-92.

[26] Resnik R. Intrauterine Growth Restriction. *Obstet Gynecol.* 2002: 99; 3.

[27] Gasbarinni.

[28] Ferguson A. Celiac disease, an eminently treatable condition, may be underdiagnosed in the United States. *Am. J. Gastroenterol* 1997;92:1252–1254.

[29] Ciacci C, Cirillo M, Auriemma G, Di Dato G, Sabbatini F, Mazzacca G Celiac disease and pregnancy outcome. *Am. J. Gastroenterol.* 1996 Apr;91(4):718-22.

[30] McCann JP, Nicholls DP, Verzin JA. Adult coeliac disease presenting with infertility. *Ulster Med. J.* 1988;57:88–89.

In: Pregnancy and Infants
Editor: Tsisana Shartava

ISBN 978-1-61209-132-7
© 2011 Nova Science Publishers, Inc.

Chapter 3

APPENDICITIS DURING PREGNANCY: A SERIOUS DISEASE AND A DIAGNOSTIC PROBLEM

L. Penninga[*] *and E. I. Penninga*

Department of Surgery CTX, Copenhagen University Hospital,
Rigshospitalet, Copenhagen, Denmark

ABSTRACT

The incidence of appendicitis during pregnancy is equal to that in the normal population. However, during pregnancy appendicitis may occur with a variety of clinical presentations, thereby causing severe diagnostic difficulties, especially during the second half of gestation. As a result, appendicitis during pregnancy is associated with an increase in perforation rate, morbidity and mortality compared to that in the normal population. In addition, it may cause pre-term birth and/or fetal loss.

[1]

[*] Corresponding author: Luit Penninga, M.D., Department of Surgery CTX, afsn. 2122, Copenhagen University Hospital, Rigshospitalet, Blegdamsvej 9, DK-2100 Copenhagen, Denmark, Email: Penninga@dadlnet.dk, Tel: (+ 45) 35451875/ 35452122. luitpenninga@hotmail.com

In this chapter we review diagnostic and treatment strategies and complications of appendicitis occuring during pregnancy

Keywords: pregnancy, appendicitis, infectious diseases

INTRODUCTION

Acute appendicitis is caused by inflammation of the vermiform apppendix and usually causes pain in the right lower abdominal quadrant, referred rebound tenderness, overlying muscle spasm and cutaneous hyperesthesia. The disease is common and occurs with an annual incidence of 0.25% in the normal population, and there is a lifetime risk for acute appendicitis of 7–9% (Rothrock). As appendicitis occurs with a high incidence in the second and third decade of life, it also occurs frequently during pregnancy, and the incidence of appendicitis during pregnancy is equal to that in the non-pregnant population (Maslovitz).

Unfortunately, appendicitis during pregnancy is associated with an increase in morbidity and mortality compared to that in the normal population, and often causes diagnostic difficulties.

In this chapter we review history, incidence, diagnostic and treatment strategies of appendicitis during pregnancy. Furthermore, we discuss maternal morbidity and mortality and the possible consequences for the fetus.

HISTORY

Berengarius Carpus, professor of surgery in Bologna and Pavia, was the first to describe the appendix in the year 1522. He spoke of a certain 'additamentum' at the end of the caecum with a breadth less than the smallest finger of the hand and a length of three inches or thereabouts (McCarthy). In 1579, Fallopius was the first to compare the appendix with a worm, and during the following centuries the anatomy of the appendix was described in more detail (McCarthy). McBurney contributed in 1889 his classical sign of the diagnosis of appendicitis, and since the 1890s the history of appendicitis consists of refinement in treatment and diagnosis. The first case of appendicitis during pregnancy was described in the 1840s by Hancock (Hancock). A century ago, Balber wrote his paper in which he reported about 200 pregnancies complicated by appendicitis (Balber). In this group there was a maternal mortality of 24% and a fetal mortality rate of 40% (Balber). Currently, a few hundred articles are found dealing with appendicitis during pregnancy. Sir Zachary Cope once stated 'the diagnosis of appendicitis (in non-pregnant patients) is usually easy'; however, he added 'but there are difficulties which need to be discussed' (Beasley). Now we know that pregnancy certainly is one of those difficulties. Borgstein and colleagues have called acute appendicitis 'a clear-cut case in men, and a guessing game in young women' (Borgstein). And we can only add that appendicitis in pregnant women is a mystery wrapped in an enigma.

INCIDENCE

Approximately 1 in 500 pregnancies is complicated by non-obstetric surgical problems (Jackson). Appendicitis is the most common non-obstetric surgical disease occuring during pregnancy, and it accounts for 25% of surgeries for non-obstetric complications in pregnancy, followed by cholecystitis and bowel obstruction (Andersen, Al-Mulhim, Dietrich). In the literature several studies describe the incidence of appendicitis during pregnancy: Maslovitz et al. reviewed 40,112 deliveries and found an incidence of appendicitis of 1/2,111 (Maslovitz); Babaknia et al. reviewed 503,496 deliveries and found an incidence of appendicitis of 1/1,500 (Babaknia); Tamir et al. reported an incidence of 1/1,400 in a review of 73,000 deliveries (Tamir); Gomez et al. found an incidence of 1/1,258 in a review of 76,608 deliveries (Gomez); Eryilmaz et al. described an incidence of 1/1,312 in a review of 31,480 deliveries (Eryilmaz); and, finally, Andersen et al. found an incidence of 1/766 pregnancies (Andersen). Some studies report that appendicitis occurs with equal frequency in each trimester of pregnancy, though others have found an overpresentation in the second trimester of pregnancy (Brown, Yilmaz). The perforation rate of appendicitis during pregnancy (43%) is much higher than that in the normal population (4–19%) (Tamir). This probably reflects the problems in diagnosing the disease, and maybe the reluctance to operate on pregnant patients. Of note, perforation of the appendix occurs twice as often in the third trimester (69%) compared to the first and second trimesters (Jackson).

ANATOMICAL APPENDICEAL DISPLACEMENT

In non-pregnant patients, classically the tenderness of acute appendicitis is localized over McBurney's point, until rupture and generalized peritonitis supervene. McBurney reports, '…I believe that in every case the seat of the greatest pain, determined by the pressure of one finger has been very exactly between an inch and a half and two inches from the anterior spinous process of the ilium on a straight line drawn from that process to the umbilicus. This may appear to be an affection of accuracy, but, so far as my experience goes this observation is correct' (McBurney, 1890). Displacement of the appendix during pregnancy from McBurney's point has been discussed in the literature: In 1932 Baer et al. performed radiological studies with barium enemas to confirm that during pregnancy anatomical displacement of the appendix occurs (Baer, Eryyilmaz). Bear's study showed that during the first trimester, the appendix had the same anatomical position as before pregnancy; however, at five months of pregnancy the appendix is placed at the iliac crest level, and rises above this level during the last trimester of pregnancy, which, according to Baer, might explain why some pregnant patients present with pain in the right upper quadrant (Baer, Eryilmaz). Seven decades later, Hodjati and colleagues performed a study in which they questioned Baer's statement that the appendix displaces during pregnancy (Hodjati). In their study, Hodjati et al. studied the position of the appendix in non-pregnant and pregnant patients undergoing appendectomy, and in pregnant patients undergoing caesarean section (Hodjati). This study showed that during surgery the appendix was located more than 8 cm from McBurney's point in 26% of the pregnant patients undergoing a ceasarean section, in 6% of the pregnant women undergoing appendectomy between 19 and 39 weeks of pregnancy and in 17% of non-pregnant patients undergoing appendectomy. From their study Hodjati concluded, opposite to Baer, that displacement of the appendix during pregnancy from McBurney's point is very limited (Baer, Hodjati).

DIAGNOSTIC FEATURES

The most common symptoms of appendicitis during pregnancy are abdominal pain (100%), nausea (88%) and vomiting (83%). Diagnosis of appendicitis during pregnancy is difficult, because many of these classical symptoms are normal during pregnancy. In addition, some patients may lack symptoms and signs of appendicitis, and diagnosis may be delayed. In general, nausea and vomiting are unreliable symptoms during pregnancy; however, the occurrence of these symptoms after the first trimester of pregnancy warrants a thorough investigation (Maslovitz). Also, new-onset abdominal pain should be taken seriously. Abdominal pain due to appendicitis during pregnancy is often less characteristic compared to abdominal pain in non-pregnant patients with appendicitis. Generally, abdominal pain is less useful in the diagnosis of appendicitis during pregnancy than abdominal pain in non-pregnant patients with appendicitis. It has been stated that all patients with appendicitis during pregnancy had had pain in the right lower quadrant of the abdomen at some period of time. Approximately 70% of patients will have rebound, referring tenderness, which is not normally encountered during regular pregnancy. One study found that patients who presented with diffuse or periumbilical pain which later migrated to the right lower quadrant of the abdomen had a significantly higher chance to have appendicitis compared to those who had a normal appendix at operation (Andersen).

Interestingly, Kurtz et al. found that a positive Bryan's sign (abdominal pain caused by shifting a pregnant uterus to the right) was the most reliable sign of appendicitis during pregnancy (Kurtz). Rectal or pelvic pain may not be present due to enlargement of the uterus which displaces the appendix away from the rectum and pelvis (Dietrich). Perforation of the appendix should be suspected in patients where the pain changes from localized tenderness to pain with a more diffuse nature. Patients who present with back, flank or leg pain or leginfection during pregnancy might have a retrocoecal located inflammed appendix (Penninga). It is generally acknowledged that diagnosing appendicitis becomes more difficult as pregnancy enhances (Maslovitz, Tracy). During pregnancy the appendix moves away from the abdominal wall due to the growing uterus. This may decrease abdominal pain and referred rebound tenderness, and increase diagnostic difficulties. In addition the pregnant uterus prevents omental isolation of the inflammatory process (Tracy, Stone).

INFECTIOUS SIGNS AND LABORATORY TESTING

Pregnancy is associated with a physiologic increase in maternal blood volume that diminishes the womens ability to demonstrate tachycardia and hypotension (Stone). Fever is not useful in diagnosing appendicitis, but an elevation in body temperature may predict perforation of the appendix (Maslovitz). During pregnancy leucocytosis may occur with an increase in neutrophils; however, neither an increase in leucocytes nor any other laboratory value has been found to be useful and reliable in diagnosing appendicitis during pregnancy (Stone, Tracy, Andersen).

RADIOLOGICAL IMAGING

Radiological imaging might be beneficial in diagnosing appendicitis during pregnancy. Ultrasonography is the preferred imaging investigation during pregnancy (Melnick). The method is cheap and safe and it has a high specificity when a pathological appendix is found. Ultrasonography has been used in large series in non-pregnant patients with a sensitivity of 75% to 89% and a specificity of 86% to 100% (Borgstein). In addition, ultrasonography is the most accurate investigation to identify a periappendiceal abcess, however it is less sensitive in identifying a ruptured appendix (Dietrich). Ultrasonography is most accurate in the first and second trimester of pregnacy, and less accurate in the third trimester of pregancy due to the enlarged uterus.

Magnetic resonance imaging (MRI) is also used in diagnosing appendicitis during pregnancy. The method has a high sensitivity and specificity, and as ultrasonography has the advantage of non-ionizing radiation, and should therefore be considered safe. In addition, unenhanced focused single-detector helical CT scanning has also been used for diagnosing appendicitis during pregnancy. This method has the advantage of limited ionizing radition compared to normal CT scanning. Although there is limited data, than unenhanced focuse single-detector helical CT scanning was found to have the same sensitivity and specificity as ultrasonography, but at the moment has no established role in the diagnostics of appendicitis during pregnancy.

TREATMENT STRATEGY AND OUTCOME

Early surgical treatment is of major importance to avoid the complications associated with perforation of the appendix. A 66% perforation rate has been reported when surgery is delayed by more than 24 hours compared to no perforations when surgical management is initiated within 24 hours after presentation (Tamir). Balber noticed this already in the beginning of the 20th century and he wrote 'The mortality of appendicitis complicating pregnancy is the mortality of delay' (Balber).

The 'early and aggressive' surgical treatment approach is also one of the reasons that appendicitis during pregnancy has a low diagnostic accuracy compared to the non-pregnant population. Twenty-five percent of the pregnant women who underwent surgery during pregnancy under the suspicion of appendicitis turn out to have a normal appendix, and in some studies even up to 50% turn out to have a normal appendix.

Pregnant patients with appendicitis can be operated on by both an open and laparoscopic approach (Al-Fozan, Carver). Possible benefits of laparoscopic surgery are decreased postoperative narcotic requirements, which might cause less fetal depression, fewer wound complications, decreased postoperative maternal hypoventilation and faster maternal recovery. Possible risks of laparoscopic surgery are premature labor (due to an increased intraabdominal pressure), decreased uterine bloodflow and uterine injury and the negative effects of a carbondioxide pneumoperitoneum (Neudecker). Several animal studies performed in the third trimester of pregnancy have shown that a carbondioxide pneumoperitoneum causes fetal acidosis and an increase in fetal heart rate and blood pressure; however, these effects seem not to be clinically significant (Hunter, Reynolds).

In general there has been a tendency to choose the open surgical approach as pregnancy advances. Lyass et al. showed nevertheless that the laparoscopic appendectomy approach is technically feasible in all trimesters of pregnancy and associated with the same known benefits of laparoscopic surgery that non-pregnant patients experience, and no maternal mortality and/or fetal loss was seen in their study (Lyass). In contrast to Lyass et al., McGory et al. found a significantly higher risk of fetal loss in patients undergoing laparoscopic appendectomy (7%) than in patients undergoing open appendectomy (3%) (McGory). During recent years, as laparoscopy has generally advanced, there has also been a trend towards more laparoscopic procedures than open procedures in patients with appendicitis during pregnancy. In patients with advanced gestation undergoing laparoscopic appendectomy it is recommended to perforate the peritoneum and to insert the first trochar under direct visualisation ('Hasson' technique) to avoid perforation of the enlarged uterus (Jackson). Alternatively, ultrasound guided trochar placement has been described to avoid uterus perforation (Jackson)

MATERNAL MORBIDITY AND MORTALITY AND FETAL LOSS

Perforation of the appendix is a major risk factor for maternal morbidity. Yilmaz et al. found a significant difference between patients with a perforated and non-perforated appendix in the rate of complications (52% vs. 17%) (Yilmaz). Earlier reports have described maternal mortality due to appendicitis during pregnancy and some years ago a maternal mortality of about 4% was common, but fortunately, in the Western world, maternal mortality has almost disappeared during the past few years.

Uncomplicated appendectomy has a 3% to 5% fetal loss rate with minimal maternal mortality. However, perforation of the appendix is associated with a 20% to 37% fetal loss rate, which has been used to justify early surgical intervention. In addition to fetal loss, appendectomy in pregnant patients causes preterm early delivery in 7–45% of the patients. Preterm delivery occurs most frequently in the first postoperative week (Mazze). Risk factors associated with preterm labor are advanced gestational age, interval between symptom onset and operation, and white blood cell count (Yilmaz). Surprisingly, one study found a preterm early delivery rate of 10% in patients undergoing surgery but with a normal appendix, compared to 11% in patients with a complicated appendicitis. The authors explain this by the fact that many of the women who were found to have a normal appendix during surgery were suffering from another disease that might have initiated preterm delivery. Threatened preterm labor might be successfully managed with tocolytic therapy (Jackson). No prophylactic effect of tocolytic treatment has been reported, but tocolytic treatment should be considered perioperatively when signs of preterm labor are present (Jackson).

CONCLUSION

Appendicitis is the most common non-obstetric surgical disease occuring during pregnancy, and it accounts for 25% of surgeries for non-obstetric complications in pregnancy.

The most common symptoms of appendicitis during pregnancy are abdominal pain, nausea and vomiting. These symptoms are all unspecific in pregnant women, as they also occur in pregnant women without appendicitis. Furthermore, infectious signs and laboratory tests are also unreliable, which makes appendicitis during pregnancy a severe diagnostic problem, and diagnosing appendicitis becomes even more difficult as pregnancy enhances. Ultrasonography is the radiological investigation of choice, and may be helpful in diagnosing appendicitis.

Early surgical treatment is of highest importance to avoid the risk of perforation, and the associated increased risk of morbidity, preterm delivery and fetal loss. Both open and laparoscopic surgical approaches can be used in pregnant patients. Appendectomy can be complicated by preterm delivery and fetal loss; however, the risk of not operating on suspected appendicitis is by far greater and justifies prompt surgery of any suspected appendicitis in pregnant patients.

Naturally, careful history, clinical and radiological investigation are still of major importance in diagnosing appendicitis during pregnancy.

REFERENCES

Al-Fozan F, Tulandi T. Safety and risks of laparoscopy in pregnancy. *Curr Opin Obstet Gynecol* 2002;14:375-9.

Al-Mulhim AA. Acute appendicitis in pregnancy: a review of 52 cases. *Int Surg* 1996;81:295-7.

Andersen B, Nielsen TF. Appendicitis in pregnancy: Diagnosis, management and complications. *Acta Obstet Gyn Scand* 1999;78:758-62.

Andersson REB. Meta-analysis of the clinical and laboratory diagnosis of appendicitis. *Br J Surg* 2004;91:28-37.

Baer JL, Reis RS, Arens RA. Appendicitis in pregnancy with changes of in position and axis of the normal appendix in pregnancy. *JAMA* 1932;16:1359-64.

Balber EA. Perforative appendicitis complicating pregnancy. *JAMA* 1908;51:1310-13.

Beasley SW. Can we improve diagnosis of acute appendicitis? *BMJ* 2000;321:907-8.

Borgstein PJ, Gordijn RV, Eijsbouts QAJ, Cuesta MA. Acute appendicitis- a clear-cut case in men, a guessing game in young women, a prospective study on the role of laparoscopy. Surg Endosc 1997; 11:923-7.

Carver TW, Antevil J, Egan JC, Brown CV. Appendectomy during early pregnancy: What is the preferred surgical approach? *Am Surg* 2005;71:

809-812.Dietrich CS III, Hill CC, Hueman M. Surgical diseases presenting during pregnancy. *Surg Clin N Am* 2008; 88:403-19.

Eryilmaz R, Sahin M, Bas G, Alimoglu O, Kaya B. Acute appendicitis during pregnancy. *Dig Surg* 2002;19:40-44

Hancock H. Disease of the appendix caeci cured by operation. *Lancet* 1848;2:380-1.

Hee P, Vikstrup L. The diagnosis of appendicitis during pregnancy and maternal and fetal outcome after appendectomy. *Int J Gyn Obstet* 1999;65:129-35.

Hodjati H, Kazerooni T. Location of the appendix in the gravid patient: a re-evaluation of the established concept. *Int J Gyn Obstet* 2003; 81:245-7.

Horrowitz M, Gomez GA, Santieesteben R, Burkett G. Acute appendicitis during pregnancy. *Arch Surg* 1985;120:1362-7.

Hunter JG, Swanstrom L, Thornburg K. Carbon dioxide pneumoperitoneum induces fetal acidosis in a pregnant ewe model. *Surg Endosc* 1995;9:272-9.

Jackson H, Granger S, Price R, Rollins M, Earle D, Richardson W, Fanelli R. Diagnosis and laparoscopic treatment of surgical diseases during pregnancy: an evidence-based review. *Surg Endosc* 2008;22:1917-27.

Kurtz RJ, Heimann TM. Comparison of open and laparoscopic treatment of acute appendicitis. *Am J Surg* 2001;182:211-4.

Lyass S, Pikarsky A, Eissenberg VH, Eichalal U, Schenker JG, Reissman P. Is laparoscopic appendectomy safe in pregnant women? *Surg Endosc* 2001;15:377-9.

Mahmoodian S. Appendicitis complicating pregnancy. *South Med J* 1992;85:19-24.

Maslovitz S, Gutman G, Lessing JB, Kupferminc MJ, Gamzu R. The significance of clinical signs and blood indices for the diagnosis of appendicitis during pregnancy. *Gyn Obstet Invest* 2003;56:189-91.

McCarthy AC. History of appendicitis vermiformis, its diseases and treatment. Lecture to the innominate society 1927. www.innominatesociety.com.

Melnick DM, Wahl WD, Dalton VK. Management of general surgical problems in the pregnant patient. *Am J Surg* 2004;187:170-180.

Mourad J, Elliot JP, Erickson L, Lisboa L. Appendicitis in pregnancy: new information that contradicts long-held clinical beliefs. *Am J Obstet Gyn* 2000;182:1027-9.

Neudecker J, Sauerland S, Neugebauer E, Bergamaschi R, Bonjer HJ, Cuschieri A, Fuchs KH, Jacobi Ch, Jansen FW, Koivusalo AM, Lacy A, McMahon MJ, Millat B, Schwenk W. European association for endoscopic surgery clinical practice guideline on the pneumoperitoneum for laparoscopic surgery. *Surg Endosc* 2002; 16:1121-43.

Penninga L, Wettergren A. Perforated appendicitis during near-term pregnancy causing necrotizing fasciitis of the lower extremity: a rare complication of a common disease. *Act Obstet Gyn Scand* 2006;85:1150-1.

Reynolds JD, Booth JV, de la Fuente S, Punnahitananda S, McMahon RL, Hopkins MB, Eubanks WS. A review of laparoscopy for non-obstetric related surgery during pregnancy. *Curr Surg* 2003;60:164-73.

Rothrock SG, Pagane J. Acute appendicitis in children: emergency department diagnosis and management. *Ann Emerg Med* 2000;36:39-51.

Stone K. Acute abdominal emergencies associated with pregnancy. *Clin Obstet Gynecol* 2002;45:553-601.

Tamir IL, Bongard FS, Klein SR. Acute appendicitis in the pregnant patient. *Am J Surg* 1990;160:571-5.

Tracy M, Fletcher HS. Appendicitis in pregnancy. *Am Surg* 2000;66:555-9.

Ueberrueck T, Koch A, Meyer L, Hinkel M, Gastinger I. Ninety-four appendectomies for suspected acute appendicitis during surgery. *World J Surg* 2004;28:508-11.

Yilmaz HG, Akgun Y, Bac B, Celik Y. Acute appendicitis in pregnancy-risk factors associated with principal outcomes: a case control study. *Int J Surg* 2007;5:192-7.

In: Pregnancy and Infants   ISBN 978-1-61209-132-7
Editor: Tsisana Shartava   © 2011 Nova Science Publishers, Inc.

Chapter 4

PROBIOTICS IN MATERNAL AND EARLY INFANT NUTRITION

Yolanda Sanz[*]

Microbial Ecophysiology and Nutrition Group.
Instituto de Agroquímica y Tecnología de Alimentos (IATA),
Consejo Superior de Investigaciones Científicas (CSIC).
PO Box 73, 46100 Burjassot, Valencia. Spain

Abstract

Fetal development is entirely dependent on the mother during pregnancy. Epidemiologic and clinical data suggest that immunologic and metabolic profiles of the pregnant uterus are responsive to mother's diet. This evidence supports the hypothesis that maternal nutrition may influence fetal programming and disease risk in the offspring. After birth, the gastrointestinal tract undergoes vast structural and functional adaptations under the stimulation of the microbiota and the diet that make possible handle with antigens and digest milk and latter solid food. The intestinal colonization process implies the activation of diverse metabolic functions either triggered by host-microbe interactions or directly

---

[*] Corresponding author: Tel.: 34 96 390 00 22; Fax: 34 96 363 63 01. E-mail: yolsanz@iata.csic.es

encoded by the genome of the microbiota (microbiome). Moreover, microbial exposure through colonization process of the newborn intestine is essential to regulate epithelial permeability and immune function, with long-term consequences on host's health. Bacterial composition and succession during the intestinal colonization process have been shown to determine susceptibility to infections and sensitization to dietary antigens. In this context, mammals seem to have a developmental window within the perinatal and postnatal period, in which the host-gut microbiota interactions are more influential in favoring later health. Probiotic and prebiotic administration has been demonstrated to be a dietary strategy that at least temporary modulates the microbiota composition and may favor a healthy status. These strategies have demonstrated moderate efficacy to reduce the risk of infections and allergic diseases early in life. In recent years, the administration of probiotics to pregnant and lactating mothers in addition to their newborns, together or not with prebiotics, has also been evaluated to extend their applications and improve effectiveness by acting in these critical developmental stages. In this type of intervention, specific probiotic strains have been demonstrated to influence gut growth and immune function in the offspring of animal models. Other studies have suggested that this dietary strategy may help to reduce the risk of atopy, infections, and metabolic disorders in humans. The current knowledge on the effectiveness and mechanisms by which the administration of probiotics to mothers and infants can positively affect early stages of development, favoring latter heath are review.

1. Introduction

The prevalence of metabolic diseases associated with obesity is increasing worldwide presumably as a result of societal changes and environmental influences. In addition, whereas hygienic conditions and medical advances have reduced the mortality from infectious diseases in most countries, immune-mediated diseases, such as allergies and autoimmune diseases, are becoming more prevalent worldwide. This has led to speculate that modern lifestyle has altered the relationship between predisposing genes and environment so as to promote development of immune and metabolic disorders, which are becoming major causes of concern and mortality in developed countries. The "hygienic hypothesis" proposed by Strachan (1989) seems to explain reasonably well the increased prevalence of immune-mediated diseases such as allergies. It is known that pregnancy favors Th2 lymphocyte development in the mother and the fetus to prevent the fetus from rejection. However, adequate exposure to microbes in early life is also essential to trigger Th1 lymphocyte development that will prevent form persistence of the Th2-biased responses in the newborn and, thereby, development of an allergic phenotype latter in life. Epidemiological and intervention studies also suggest that diet and exposure to microbes influence the metabolic and immunologic profiles of the pregnant uterus and the risk of immune and metabolic disease development in the offspring (Yajnik et al., 2006; Barker et al., 2007, Ege et al., 2008). A number of preclinical and clinical intervention studies based on nutritional restrictions, high-fat diets and functional ingredient supplementation (e.g. polyunsaturated fatty acids and probiotics) during pregnancy have revealed a close relationship between mother's diet and infant's health (Herrera et al., 2002; Church et al., 2009) supporting the fetal programming hypothesis proposed by Barker et al. (2007). Therefore, the interplay between both heredity and environmental factors (diet, microbes and xenobiotics) seems to affect every stage of development from conception to early postnatal period with potential long-term effects in child and adult health. Thus, it can be anticipated that further research on the convergence of both theories "hygienic" and "fetal programming" will better explain the current disease trends.

The intestinal microbiota develops an array of physiological roles within the human body, shaping its metabolic abilities and immune responses. The intestinal colonization process of the newborn intestine seems to be a particularly relevant process to the infant's health (Sanz et al., 2008a). The microbiota provides novel metabolic capacities and also regulates host gene expression to favor both host and microbe survival. In addition, microbial exposure through colonization of the newborn intestine is essential to fully boost the immune system and to regulate permeability, with long-term consequences on health. Microbiota acquisition and succession in the newborn's intestine has been shown to determine susceptibility to infections and sensitization to dietary antigens (Kalliomaki et al.2007). An adequate colonization process may be achieved by dietary intervention based on probiotic and prebiotic administration to the infants. However, while probiotic administration seems to provide only temporary changes in a fully developed gut ecosystem, a practically sterile newborn intestine seems to be more amenable to manipulation by dietary strategies. Evidence on the transmission of bacteria from the mother to the neonate has also encouraged the administration of probiotic-based products to the mother during the perinatal period and lactation to favor infants gut colonization. This practice also seems to provide additional benefits by influencing, for instance, breast-milk composition and immune functions on the mother-fetal interface. Therefore, the incorporation of probiotic-based products into both maternal and infant nutrition is being investigated as a novel dietary approach to reduce disease risk in the light of both the hygienic and the fetal programming hypotheses. The current knowledge on the effectiveness and mechanisms by which probiotics could positively act at early stages of development favoring latter heath are review and discussed in the following sections.

2. Microbial Acquisition and Evolution in the Newborn Intestine

Infants are born with a practically sterile intestine that is rapidly colonized after birth. The colonization during the first 12-24 hours of life is characterized by the presence of higher levels of facultative anaerobes (e.g. *Enterobacteriaceae*, *Enterococcus*, and *Streptococcus*) than strict anaerobic bacteria (e.g. *Bifidobacterium*, *Bacteroides* and *Clostridium)*, but these proportions are reversed within a week after birth when an anaerobic environment is established (Mackie et al., 1999). The infant microbiota, which is characterized by low diversity and instability, evolves into a typical adult microbiota over the first 24 months of life. Then, it becomes more stable and diverse and seems to be unique for each individual (Zoetendal et al., 1998). The acquisition and succession of the gut microbiota depend on diverse external and internal host factors. External factors include the gestational age, intake of medicines, microbial load from the environment, mode of delivery, mother's microbiota, number of siblings and type of feeding and solid diet. Internal factors include the gastrointestinal physiology that influences peristalsis, bile acid concentrations and gastrointestinal pH, as well as other genotypic determinants of gut colonization, which are less well characterized (Björkstén, 2006; Sanz et al., 2008a).

Gestational age has been suggested to influence the gut microbiota, particularly when comparing preterm and full-term infants due to differences in exposure to environmental microbes and antibiotics. In general, colonization of the intestine with beneficial bacteria is delayed in preterm infants and the number of potentially pathogenic bacteria is higher than in full-term healthy infants. Analyses of the microbial succession patterns during the first 4 weeks of life revealed that *E. coli, Enterococcus,* and *Klebsiella pneumoniae* were common in the microbiota of hospitalized preterm infants, but not in that full-term infants. In addition, *Bifidobacterium* species were not detected preterm infants in contrast to what found in full-term infants (Schwiertz et al., 2003). The microbial patterns of preterm infants also became more similar to one another over time, supporting the hypothesis that environmental factors influence the initial colonization of the newborn intestine. Other studies have also associated hospitalization and prematurity with higher prevalence and counts of *Clostridium difficile* (Penders et al., 2006). The fact that many preterm infants receive prophylactic antibiotics at birth may affect the intestinal colonization (Westerbeek et al., 2006) and reductions in the numbers of *Bifidobacterium* and *Bacteroides* have been associated with this clinical practice (Penders et al., 2006).

The mother's microbiota (vaginal, intestinal, oral and cutaneous microbiota) also influence the infant's gut colonization (Mackie et al., 1999). During birth, exposure to the mother's vaginal and intestinal microbiota due to the proximity between the birth canal and the anus is likely to influence the initial colonizers of the newborn intestine. After birth, cutaneous and oral mother's microbiota will also be easily transferred to the newborn by kissing and sucking (Lindberg et al., 2004). In particular, a relation between the infant's microbiota and type of delivery has been inferred in diverse studies. This has partly been explained by the lack of initial contact of infants delivered by caesarean section with the mother's vaginal microbiota. Microbes from the vaginal canal and anus area seem to be able to enter the mouth and stomach of vaginally delivered infants within few minutes after birth. However, the vaginal microbiota seems to settle-down in the newborn intestine less easily than the maternal intestinal microbiota (Mackie et al., 1999). In general, caesarean-delivered infants experience some delay in bacterial colonization, and their microbiota present aberrancies that can last for up to 1 year (Adlerberth et al., 2006). Some studies showed that the fecal microbiota of caesarean-delivered infants harbors significantly fewer *Bacteroides* species compared with that of vaginally delivered infants (Grönlund et al., 2000; Adlerberth et al., 2006), which was suggested to be associated with maturation of humoral immunity (Grönlund et al., 2000). Bifidobacteria colonization was also shown to be delayed and reached lower levels in the caesarean delivered infants than in the vaginally delivered infants (Chen et al., 2007). Another study also revealed that the microbiota of the caesarean delivered group was less diverse, in terms of bacteria species, than the microbiota of the vaginally delivered group after 3 days of life (Biasucci et al., 2008). Moreover, *Bifidobacterium* species were absent in the microbiota of caesarean delivered infants, while *B. longum* and *B. catenulatum* group were predominant in that of vaginally delivered neonates (Biasucci et al., 2008). In addition, mode of delivery seems to have significant effects on immunological functions of the infant, probably via its influence on gut microbiota colonization (Huurre et al. 2008a). At 1 month of age, the total gut bacterial counts in feces were higher in vaginally delivered infants than in caesarean section delivered infants, mainly due to higher bifidobacterial counts. In contrast, the total number of IgA-, IgG- and IgM-secreting cells was lower in infants vaginally delivered than in those delivered by caesarean section during the first year of life, possibly reflecting excessive antigen exposure across the vulnerable gut barrier of the last group (Huurre et al., 2008a). In a large study of 1032 infants at 1 month of age, those born through caesarean section had lower numbers of *Bifidobacterium* and *Bacteroides*, whereas they were more often colonized with *Clostridium difficile*, compared with vaginally born infants (Penders et al., 2006).

An increased number of siblings can also be related to the newborn microbiota as it implies an increased microbial exposure by direct contact with the newborn. In some studies, infants with older siblings had slightly higher numbers of bifidobacteria compared with infants without siblings (Penders et al., 2006) but this was not demonstrated in all studies (Ahrné et al., 2005).

The type of milk-feeding is regarded as one of the major environmental factors influencing gut colonization early in life. In general, the *Bifidobacterium* genus is dominant in the microbiota of breast-fed infants (up to 90% of the total fecal bacteria), while a more-diverse adult-like microbiota is characteristic of formula-fed infants (Salminen & Isolauri, 2006). A large-scale population study has showed that exclusively formula-fed infants were more often colonized with *E. coli, C. difficile, Bacteroides* and *Lactobacillus*, compared with breast-fed infants (Penders et al., 2006). A delay in *Bifidobacterium* species colonization in formula-fed compared with breast-fed babies has also been shown by other authors (Favier et al., 2003). In addition, differences in *Bifidobacterium* species composition as a function of the type of milk-feeding have been reported. Some authors showed that *B. breve* was predominant in breast-fed infants, whereas *B. longum* and *B. adolescentis* were more often present in formula-fed infants (Mitsuoka & Kaneuchi, 1977; Mevissen-Verhag et al., 1987). More recently, another comparative molecular analysis of the infant's microbiota has showed that breast-fed infants had significantly higher levels of total *Bifidobacterium* and *B. breve*, and lower levels of *B. adolescentis* and *B. catenulatum* than formula-fed infants, resembling the bifidobacterial populations of the adult microbiota (Haarman & Knol, 2005). However, other authors have not found significant differences in *Bifidobacterium* species composition a function of type of feeding (Favier et al., 2003). Breast milk seems to be a source of commensal bacteria to the infant's gut, including *Staphylococcus, Lactobacillus* and *Bifidobacterium* (Martín et al., 2008). *B. breve, B. adolescentis* and *B. bifidum* have been isolated from human milk in culture medium and, therefore, at least these species could be transferred alive to the newborn via breast-feeding. Breast-milk bifidobacteria composition was also analyzed by real-time PCR showing that *B. longum* was the most widely found species followed by *B. animalis, B. bifidum* and *B. catenulatum*; however, these data are based on DNA detention not on viability (Gueimonde et al., 2007). Moreover, allergic mothers have been shown to have significantly lower amounts of bifidobacteria in breast-milk compared with non-allergic mothers and their infants have concurrently lower counts of bifidobacteria in feces. Therefore, the maternal health status could alter the counts of bifidobacteria in breast-milk and influence the infants' fecal *Bifidobacterium* levels (Grönlund et al., 2007). Breast-milk also contains prebiotic substances (oligosaccharides), which stimulate the growth of *Bifidobacterium* and are one of the major *bifidogenic* factors (González et al., 2008). In fact, *Bifidobacterium longum* biovar *infantis* ATCC 15697, an isolate from the infant gut, preferentially consumes small mass oligosaccharides, which represent 63.9% of the total human milk oligosaccharides available (LoCascio et al., 2007). Accordingly, the complete genome sequence of this strain reflects a competitive ability to utilize milk-borne molecules, which lack a nutritive value to the neonate (Sela et al., 2008). Breast-milk contains other bioactive factors, such as secretory IgA, lactoferrin and a range of cytokines, which have a remarkable effect on the development of the neonatal microbiota and mucosal immunity. In particular, IgA supplied by maternal milk has been shown to sequester commensal bacteria in the mice neonatal intestine, thereby delaying active development of IgA production (Kramer & Cebra, 1995), while the decline in maternal IgA supply increases intestinal bacterial colonization in pups (Inoue et al., 2005). In formula-fed infants no detectable levels of fecal IgA were found during the first 10 days of life, which might partially explain the development of a more-diverse microbiota in these infants at an early age (Bakker-Zierikzee et al., 2006).

Few studies have demonstrated a relationship between the genotype and the gut microbial colonization process so far. Similarity between fecal bacterial DNA profiles of monozygotic twins was shown to be significantly greater than that between profiles of unrelated individuals (Zoetendal et al., 2001). Furthermore, the DNA profiles of the fecal microbiota of monozygotic twins were also significantly more similar than those of dizygotic twins (Stewart et al., 2005). It can be anticipated, that the host genotype may influence for instance the repertory of mucins, acting as bacterial adhesion sites in the intestinal mucosa, and the immune response, which altogether will restrict or allow the colonization of certain micro-organisms (Björkstén, 2006; Sanz et al., 2008a). However, some studies suggest that the shared environment influences the gut microbiota to a higher extent than the genotype (Palmer et al., 2007). In particular, studies on the evolution of mammals and their gut microbes by metagenomic approaches pointed out that the acquisition of a new diet is a fundamental driver for changes in gut bacterial diversity (Ley et al., 2008). This scientific evidence supports the hypothesis that dietary intervention strategies may play a critical role in health and disease prevention, probably via modulation of the gut microbiota and its functions. Consequently, probiotic and prebiotic based nutritional strategies could play a primary role in this field, which will become a reality as we improve our understanding of the roles of intestinal bacteria in the human body.

3. Roles of the Intestinal Microbiota in Host Physiology and Immunity During the Early Postnatal Period

3.1. Roles of the Intestinal Microbiota in Host Physiology and Metabolism

The anatomy and physiology of the intestine depend on the interactions between the microbiota and the diet with the host epithelium, mucosal immune system and microvasculature (Hooper et al., 2002). After birth, the gastrointestinal tract undergoes vast structural and functional adaptations to be able to initially digest mother's milk and later solid food. During the early suckling period, the morphological and functional gut development is reflected in a rapid intestinal growth and increased expression of digestive enzymes such as lactase. At weaning period, crypt hyperplasia and an increased expression of maltase, sucrase, and pancreatic trypsin also denote vast changes of the gastrointestinal tract to digest a more complex diet. It is known that the gut microbiota plays an important role in these gastrointestinal maturation processes from gnotobiology studies (Fåk et al., 2008). In germ-free animals the intestinal weight and surface area are decreased, the intestinal villi are thinner, and the shape of enterocytes is abnormal compared with conventionally raised mice (Berg, 1996). In contrast, the mecum is much larger in germ-free animals due to mucus and fiber accumulation and subsequent water retention when compared with conventionally raised animals (McCracken & Lorenz, 2001). In preterm formula-fed animal, the administration of specific bacteria immediately after birth limits the formula-induced mucosal atrophy, dysfunction, and pathogen load in preterm neonates. This strategy also increases the intestinal weight, mucosa proportion, villus height, RNA integrity, and brush border aminopeptidase A and N activities, reflecting the role of bacteria in intestinal physiology (Siggers et al., 2008).

It is known that intestinal microbiota develops an important biochemical activity within the human body by both providing additional metabolic capacities encoded by the microbiome to the host (Gill et al., 2006) and by regulating diverse aspects of cellular differentiation and gene expression via host-microbe interactions (Hooper et al., 2002).

The intestinal microbiota provides additional metabolic capacities, involved in the utilization of no digestible carbohydrates and host-derived glycoconjugates (e.g. chondroitin sulphate, mucin, hyaluronate and heparin), deconjugation and dehydroxylation of bile acids, cholesterol reduction and biosynthesis of vitamins (K and B group), isoprenoids and amino acids (e.g. lysine and threonine) (Hooper et al., 2002, Gill et al., 2006). In particular, the ability of the commensal microbiota to utilize complex dietary polysaccharides, that would otherwise be inaccessible to humans, may contribute to the ability of the host to harvest energy from the diet, which may represent 10% of the daily energy supply (Sanz et al., 2008b). In addition, *B. thetaiotaomicron,* a prominent commensal bacteria, has been shown to have ability to hydrolyze host-derived glycans and influence the nature of those produced by the host by increasing expression of fucosylated ones to favor its own colonization (Hooper et al., 2001).

The commensal microbiota also induces expression of genes involved in the processing and absorption of dietary carbohydrates and complex lipids in the host (Hooper et al., 2001; Bäckhed et al., 2004). For instance, ileal expression of a monosaccharide transporter (Na+/glucose co-transporter) was induced in *B. thetaiotaomicron* mono-colonized mice, which would lead to increasing the absorption of dietary monosaccharides and short-chain fatty acids and, thereby, promoting *the novo* synthesis of lipids in the liver (Hooper et al., 2001). The colonization of germ-free mice by conventional microbiota also increased liver expression of key enzymes (acetyl-CoA carboxylase and fatty acid synthase) involved in the *de novo* fatty acid biosynthetic pathways, and transcriptional factors (ChREBP and SREBP-1) involved in hepatocyte lipogenic responses to insulin and glucose (Bäckhed et al., 2004). In addition, the colonization reduced the levels of circulating fasting-induced adipose factor (Fiaf) and the skeletal muscle and liver levels of phosphorylated AMP-activated protein kinase, which altogether contribute to fat storage (Bäckhed, et al., 2007). The colonization of germ-free mice by *B. thetaiotaomicron* also increased the expression of other components involved in the host's lipid absorption machinery, including a pancreatic-lipase related protein that hydrolyzes triacylglycerols, a cytosolic fatty acid binding protein (L-FABP) involved in intracellular trafficking of fatty acids, and the apolipoprotein A-IV that mediates export of triacylglycerols re-synthesized in the enterocyte (Hooper et al., 2001). The expression of genes involved in absorption of dietary metal ions was also modified by the microbiota, which for instance induced the expression of a high affinity copper transporter in the epithelium (Hooper et al, 2001). Furthermore, the colonization of the intestinal mucosa was also implicated in the regulation of the under laying microvasculature and angiogenesis (Stappenbeck, et al., 2002).

3.2. Roles of the Intestinal Microbiota in Host Immunity

An adequate colonization process of the newborn intestine by commensal bacteria provides substantial stimuli for the correct maturation of gut barrier function and immunity during the postnatal period, whereas alterations in this process may precede the development of immune-mediated diseases (Sanz et al., 2008a). After birth, the gastrointestinal system is immature and relatively permeable to macromolecules, but this high permeability declines with age until a more mature gut barrier is established at weaning. Commensal bacteria regulate intestinal permeability and, thus, contribute to the physical barrier that prevents the entry of harmful agents. For instance, some commensal and probiotic bacteria are able to protect against leakage of tight-junctions and alterations in cytoskeleton integrity associated with infections, stress and inflammatory conditions (Lutgendorff et al., 2008). The gut microbiota also influences the secretion of various protective substances by epithelial cells such as mucins and antimicrobial peptides. Commensal bacteria regulate mucin gene expression by goblet cells, modifying the glycosylation pattern and the expression of MUC-2 and MUC-3 genes, which may influence bacterial adhesion and colonization (Mack et al., 2003; Freitas et al., 2005; Caballero-Franco et al., 2007). The secretion of antimicrobial peptides (defensins, C-type lectins and angiogenins) by intestinal Paneth cells can also be stimulated by Gram-negative and Gram-positive (Ayabe et al., 2000;

Hooper et al., 2003; Cash et al., 2006; Vaishnava et al., 2008), constituting mechanism whereby commensal bacteria influence gut ecology and regulate non-specific intestinal defenses during the postnatal period.

Microbial colonization of germ-free animals also has an important impact on postnatal development of mucosal and systemic immunity. The gut-associated lymphoid tissue (GALT) is immature in germ-free mice, showing a reduced content of the lamina propria CD4+ T cells, IgA producing B cells and intraepithelial T cells. Systemic immunity is also affected by the absence of the microbiota and germ-free mice have decreased serum immunoglobulin levels and smaller mesenteric lymph nodes and spleens (Hrncir et al., 2008). The interaction of the gut microbiota with the GALT contributes to the production of secretory-IgA, modulation of cytokine and chemokine release, and development of balanced T helper (h) 1/Th2 responses and oral tolerance to innocuous antigens (Sanz et al., 2008a). The immune system should be regulated to such a way that can mount an effective innate and acquired mucosal and humoral response to eliminate the invader organism, but avoid collateral tissue damage and overreactions to harmless microbes and antigens. One of the key events in the regulation of appropriate immune responses is the differentiation between pathogenic and commensal bacteria. This is achieved by pattern-recognition receptors (Toll-like receptors [TLRs] and Nod-like receptors [NLRs]) expressed in epithelial and antigen presenting cells (macrophages and dendritic cells [DC]), which act as sentinels sensing the environment and activating defenses in face to danger (Winkler et al., 2007). In particular TLR-signaling commonly leads to the activation of nuclear factor kappa B (NF-κB) transcription pathway, with up regulation of major histocompatibility complexes and co stimulatory proteins, production of pro-inflammatory cytokines and chemokines (TNF-α, IL-1β, and IL-8), and recruitment of other immune cells. Signaling through TLR also stimulates the maturation of DCs with enhanced ability to present antigens and activate T cells, T-cell co-stimulatory molecules (CD80 and CD86) and other activation markers. T-cell differentiation into Th 1, Th2 or regulatory T cells (Tregs) is also thought to depend on the type of TLRs involved (Winkler et al., 2007). Th1 responses are usually associated with inflammatory reactions and clearance of pathogenic bacteria and virus, Th2 responses with allergic responses and parasite clearance, and Tregs (Th3 and Thr1) are essential in preventing overreactions (Sanz et al., 2007a). Some of the mechanism by which commensal bacteria, unlikely pathogens, have been shown to down-regulate pro-inflammatory responses include: (i) the inhibition of the NF-κB, either by regulating the nuclear export of NF-κB subunit relA (Kelly et al.,

2004) or by inhibiting the IκB ubiquitination (Neish et al., 2000); (ii) the inhibition of TLR2-driven activation of NF-κB via NOD signaling (Watanabe et al., 2008); (iii) the regulation of TLR expression and up-regulation of the negative regulator Tollip protein (Otte et al., 2004; Solano-Aguilar et al., 2008), (iv) the down-regulation of the expression of pro-inflammatory type I IFN related genes (Munakata et al., 2008), and (v) the induction of immunoregulatory cytokine production (IL-10 and TGF-β1) and Tregs (Hrncir et al., 2008).

4. Influence of the Mother's Diet and Environmental Exposures in Fetal Programming and Infant's Health

Scientific evidence indicates that the diet influence the fetal-maternal relationships with consequences on development and long-term health. The quality of the maternal diet during pregnancy has been related to offspring's risk of developing allergies, type 1 and type 2 diabetes, arteriosclerosis, cardiovascular disease and obesity (Bertino et al., 2006; Lamb et al., 2008; Yates et al., 2008). Pregnancy is seen as a period of maximum sensitivity to dietary influences since diverse organs and systems are in development in the fetus. In particular, immune and metabolic functions of the fetus are dependent on the mother and probably the refinement of their functions is already initiated inside the uterus.

Successful pregnancy requires immunologic changes characterized by a dominance of Th2 and regulatory T cell effector responses in both mother and fetus, which help to maintain pregnancy and avoid the rejection of the immunologically incompatible fetus; however the persistence of this immune polarization favors the development of a long-lasting atopic phenotype latter in life (Calder et al., 2006; Kalliomaki et al., 2007). At least during the third trimester of human pregnancy, fetal T cells are able to mount antigen-specific responses to environmental and food-derived antigens and antigen-specific T cells are detectable in cord blood, indicating fetus sensitization in uterus (Calder et al., 2006). For example, the fetus mounted an immune response to rubella antigens whose mothers were infected with rubella during pregnancy. In infected fetuses, total IgM and IgA concentrations rose significantly, and rubella virus-specific IgM and IgA antibodies were detected as early as week 22 of pregnancy (Grangeot-Keros et al., 1988). A recent investigation has determined the relationships of cord blood immunoglobulin E (IgE) with maternal health conditions before and during pregnancy, showing inverse associations of cord blood IgE to seasonal allergens with positive maternal records for *Toxoplasma gondii* and rubella virus infections. Therefore, maternal immune responses to certain pathogenic antigens may influence atopic sensitization in the fetus (Ege et al., 2008). Studies of the incidence of human pathogenic bacteria and virus (cytomegalovirus and herpes simplex virus type 1 and 2) in biopsy samples from the placenta and decidua of women with healthy pregnancies by PCR, showed that 38% of placental samples were positive for the selected microorganisms. Moreover, analyses of immunoglobulin G isolated from the placenta support the hypothesis that immune responses suppress cytomegalovirus reactivation in the presence of pathogenic bacteria at the maternal-fetal interface, suggesting that at least microbial DNA at the placenta may drive immune responses (McDonagh et al., 2004). *Bifidobacterium* spp. and *L. rhamnos*us have also been identified in human placenta by quantitative real-time PCR recently (Satokari et al., 2008). Although cultivable bacteria were not detected, the possibility that the fetus is exposed to bacterial components (e.g. DNA) via the mother's placenta during pregnancy can not be disregarded. In particular, the unmethylated CpG oligodeoxynucleotide motifs of bacterial DNA are known to activate Toll-like receptor 9 and subsequently trigger Th-1-type immune responses; this could be one of the mechanisms involved in programming the infant's immune development during fetal life (Lee et al., 2006). A recent study has also found a close relationship between maternal and cord-blood specific IgE patterns to cow milk suggesting that the immune system can be stimulated by food allergens before birth (Bertino et al., 2006). Another study analyzed whether asthma prevention could start even earlier, before conception, by transfer of immunologic tolerance from the mother to the offspring in animal models (Polte et al., 2008). The offspring of naive mothers had an asthma-like phenotype, while the offspring of tolerized mice with oral ovalbumin before conception were completely protected. The levels of allergen-specific IgG were increased in the sera of the mother, fetus, pup and breast milk, indicating their involvement in tolerance transfer from mother to the offspring (Polte et al., 2008). In addition, environmental exposure of the pregnant woman to microbes has been related to the allergic predisposition of the neonate. Therefore, the fetal immune system during the perinatal period can be responsive to environmental challenges (microbes or dietary compounds), which may not be longer effective in adulthood to prevent disease.

Dietary supply of nutrients during conception and pregnancy may also influence the development of the fetus and offspring, and the risk of suffering metabolic diseases. Maternal obesity from exogenous origin and both maternal hyperglycemia and hyperlipidemia are thought to contribute to the development of metabolic disorders in the offspring. Studies on the effect of chronic high-fat diet on the development of fetal metabolic systems in nonhuman primates showed that a developing fetus is highly vulnerable to excess of dietary lipids, independent of maternal diabetes and/or obesity, and that the risk of pediatric non-alcoholic fatty liver disease may increased by exposure to this diet (McCurdy et al., 2009). Scientific evidence has also indicated that prenatal nutrition may affect dietary preferences and may contribute to more atherogenic lipid profiles later in life. Studies in animal models have suggested that fetal undernutrition can predispose to hypercholesterolemia and metabolic disorders directly by programming cholesterol metabolism and indirectly influencing lifestyle choices. For example, pregnant women exposed to famine in early gestation were twice as likely to consume a high-fat diet and also seemed to be less physically active; although this result did not reach statistical significance (Lussana et al., 2008).

5. Probiotic and Prebiotic Concepts and Applications

The colonization process of the newborn intestine is considered critical to the health status and risk of developing disease in early and later stages of life. Therefore, improving the characteristics of the gut microbiota particularly in the prerinatal and postnatal periods is foreseen as a strategy to prevent the onset of disease (Sanz et al., 2008a). This could be achieved by the administration of probiotics, prebiotics or their combination (synbiotics). Probiotics are defined as live microbes that when administered in adequate amounts confer a health benefit to the host [FAO/WHO, 2002]. Prebiotics are non-digestible dietary ingredients that allow changes, in the composition and/or activity of the gastrointestinal microbiota that confer benefits on the host's health (Roberfroid, 2007). The genus *Bifidobacterium* is the predominant in the intestinal tract of infants, represents about 3-7% of the fecal microbiota of healthy adults and is associated with beneficial effects on health (Sanz et al., 2007a). The genus *Lactobacillus* also inhabits the gastrointestinal tract and some species are widely used in diverse food fermentations. These features have made these two bacterial genera the most attractive as probiotics for human consumption (Sanz et al., 2007b). Currently, these are incorporated into functional foods in the form of fermented milks, infant formula, cheese, ice cream and juices, and in pharmaceutical preparations. Milk fermented products constitute the best vehicle for probiotic bacteria since this matrix allows maintenance of viability and metabolic activity (Sanz et al., 2007b). Galacto-oligosaccharides and inulin-derivatives are the prebiotics most commonly commercialized in Europe (Haarman & Knol, 2005; Kelly, 2008). They are mainly added to infant formula to promote the prevalence of a microbiota composition similar to that resulting from breast-feeding during both milk-feeding and the weaning period. The administration of these prebiotic infant formulas has demonstrated to increase the total amount of fecal bifidobacteria and modify the *Bifidobacterium* species composition, resembling that of breast-fed infants, when compared with infants receiving conventional formula (Haarman & Knol, 2005; Scholtens et al., 2006).

The immaturity of the immune system and the increased epithelial permeability of the newborn intestine under lack of appropriate microbial stimulation seem to partly explain the increased prevalence of immune-mediated diseases in developed countries, such as allergies (the hygienic hypothesis). Initial attempts to control the development of allergies and food intolerance were based on the avoidance of the allergen in the diets, but the results were not satisfactory regarding long-term prevention. In recent years, novel methods including probiotic supplementation have been evaluated to counteract the immunological and gut mucosal barrier dysfunction associated with these disorders, and to strengthen endogenous defense mechanisms. Moreover, while the administration of probiotics to adults with a fully developed intestinal microbiota produces only temporary colonization of the bacteria, the newborn intestine is more amenable to dietary and probiotic manipulation in the early postnatal period. Therefore, the use of probiotics early in life has been evaluated for preventing allergies, repeated infections and necrotizing enterocolitis, and provided some promising results in preclinical trials in animals (Siggers et al., 2008) and in clinical trials in humans (Lodinova-Zadnikova et al., 2003). A step beyond this concept has been the administration of probiotics, together or not with prebiotics, to pregnant women and their infants to influence both the intrauterine and postnatal development of the newborn, relaying on the "fetal programming theory". These strategies are currently under investigation to prevent both immune and metabolic disorders with the hope that they will influence more effectively the infant's health from conception onwards.

6. Influence of Probiotic Intake by Mother and Offspring in Animals

Several studies have showed that exposure of pregnant mothers to specific probiotic bacteria prior to parturition and during lactation influences diverse physiological functions in the intestine of the offspring. The administration of the probiotic *Lactobacillus plantarum* 299v in the drinking water to pregnant and lactating rat dams until their pups had reached an age of 14 days resulted in the colonization of both mothers and pups gut by the bacterial strain and influenced gut growth and function of pups (Fåk et al., 2008). The small intestine, pancreas, spleen and liver weighed more in the probiotic colonized pups than in the control pups. The probiotic colonized pups also showed decreased gut permeability as compared to the control pups (Fåk et al., 2008). Nevertheless, the effects derived from maternal probiotic intake and their transmission to the offspring as such could be questioned since the administration of the probiotic through the drinking water could have facilitated direct contact and acquisition of the probiotic strain by the pups. The effects of *L. rhamnosus* GG supplementation to female mice intragastrically every day before conception, during pregnancy and lactation (perinatal supplementation group) or only during pregnancy (prenatal supplementation group) on the development of experimental allergic asthma in the offspring have also been investigated recently (Blümer et al., 2007). Intestinal colonization with *L. rhamnosus* GG was observed in mother mice, but not in the offspring. In spite of that, a reduced expression of TNF-α, IFN-γ, IL-5 and IL-10 was observed in splenic mononuclear cells of mice derived from mothers perinatally supplemented with *L. rhamnosus* GG. Moreover, allergic airway and peribronchial inflammation and goblet cell hyperplasia were significantly reduced in offspring of prenatally or perinatally mothers supplemented with *L. rhamnosus* GG as compared to control mice. Exposure to *L. rhamnosus* GG during pregnancy shifted the placental cytokine expression pattern with a markedly increased TNF-α level. Thus, the results suggest that this probiotic strain may exert beneficial effects on the development of experimental allergic asthma, when applied in a very early phase of life and that the effects are partly mediated via the placenta by induction of pro-inflammatory cell signals (Blümer et al., 2007). In this regard, it is worthwhile mentioning, that DNA from *Bifidobacterium* spp. and *L. rhamnosus* has been identified in human placenta and its influence on transmission of immune signals to the fetus through this route cannot be disregarded as described in the next section (Satokari et al., 2008).

The oral supplementation of *Bifidobacterium animalis* subsp *lactis* Bb12 (Bb12) to sows during gestation and to their piglets for 91 days since birth led to the establishment of increased numbers of the probiotic in the piglets' proximal colon compared to placebo-treated piglets born to placebo-treated sows, Bb12-treated sows, or piglets born to placebo sows but treated with Bb12 immediately after birth. This effect was associated with a significant up-regulation of TLR-9 expression in proximal colon, but neither of TLR2 nor TLR4. This result suggests that exposure of the mother to Bb12 influenced both Bb12 load in the piglet in the presence of continuous daily feeding and significantly affected the host innate immune system development (Solano-Aguilar et al., 2008).

The protective mechanisms of action of *L. rhamnosus* GG against atopic dermatitis development have also been studied in a mice model (NC/Nga mice) of human atopic dermatitis (Sawada et al., 2007). Maternal and infant mice were fed with food containing or not containing heat-treated *L. rhamnosus* GG during pregnancy and breastfeeding, and after weaning. While control NC/Nga mice raised under an air-uncontrolled condition spontaneously manifested typical skin lesions, probiotic feeding inhibited the onset and development of atopic skin lesions and reduced the numbers of mast cells and eosinophils in the affected skin sites. The probiotic-fed mice also showed a significant increase in plasma IL-10 levels and in the IL-10 mRNA expression in both Peyer's patches and mesenteric lymph nodes compared with control mice. However, there was no significant difference in the proportion of splenic CD4(+)CD25(+) regulatory T cells between the probiotic-fed mice and the control mice. Therefore, the ability of the probiotic *L. rhamnosus* GG to delay the onset and suppress the development of atopic dermatitis was mediated by a strong induction of IL-10 in intestinal lymphoid organs and al systemic level.

Although the number of preclinical studies is limited, the accumulated scientific evidence suggests that maternal probiotic intake, particularly when occurring prior and after birth, influences the development of the offspring, although these effects are not always correlated with the ability of the probiotic to colonize the offspring intestine. Moreover, animal studies also support a role for maternal probiotic intake in disease prevention and, particularly, in atopic disease.

7. Influence of Probiotic by Mothers and Infants in Humans

7.1. Influence of Maternal Probiotic Intake in the Intestinal Microbiota of the Infants

The clinical trials carried out to investigate the effects of the oral administration of probiotic bacteria only to the pregnant women or to both pregnant woman and their infants on children physiology and health are summarized in table 1. A pilot study including six women, who were taking *L. rhamnosus* GG during late pregnancy but discontinued its consumption at the time of delivery, was carried out to evaluate the influence of probiotic intake in their children, who did not received the probiotic after birth (Schultz et al., 2004). The results showed that temporary colonization of the infant's gut with *L. rhamnosus* GG was possible by colonizing the pregnant mother before delivery and that this colonization was stable for as long as 6 months, and could persist for up to 24 months (Schultz et al., 2004). Further studies showed that the administration of *L. rhamnosus* GG to mothers, 4 weeks before and 3 weeks after delivery, induced specific changes in the transfer and initial establishment of bifidobacteria in the neonates (Gueimonde et al, 2006). Infants whose mothers received *L. rhamnosus* GG showed a significantly higher presence of *B. breve* and lower of *B. adolescentis* than those from the placebo group at 5 days of age. *B. adolescentis* prevalence in the mother before delivery was correlated with its presence in the infant samples at 5 and 1 month and similar effects were detected for *B. catenulatum* and *B. longum* at 1 month; although these effects were only significant in the placebo group. Altogether these results suggest the transfer of bacteria from the mother to the newborn. However, *L. rhamnosus* GG consumption also increased the bifidobacterial diversity in infants at 3 weeks and reduced the similarity of *Bifidobacterium* microbiota between mother and infant (Gueimonde et al., 2006), which partly contradicts the evidence on the transference of fecal microbiota from the mother to the newborn.

Table 1. Outcomes of maternal and infant probiotic intake in humans

Probiotic/prebiotics/Diet	Administration pattern	Trial outcome	Reference
L. rhamnosus GG	Intake by women at late pregnancy but not after delivery	Probiotic colonization of the infant's gut	Schultz et al., 2004
L. rhamnosus GG	Intake by women 4 weeks before and 3 weeks after delivery	Changes in bifidobacteria transfer and establishment of in the neonates	Gueimonde et al, 2006
Fermented milk/ yogurt bacteria	Oral intake by women at 34 weeks pregnancy or vaginal application from first trimester onwards	Reduction of genital infection risk	Othman et al., 2007
Lactobacillus casei DN114401	Intake by women 6 weeks before delivery and during 6 weeks of lactation	Natural killer cell increase in mother's peripheral blood and decrease of TNF-α in breast-milk Decrease of gastrointestinal episodes in infants	Ortiz-Andrellucchiet al., 2008
L. rhamnosus GG and LC705 *Bifidobacterium breve* Bb99 *Propionibacterium freudenreichii* ssp *shermanii* and galacto-oligosaccharides	Probiotic intake by women at allergy risk during the last month of pregnancy and by their infants until age of 6 months plus a prebiotic	Increased resistance to respiratory infections in children during 2 years A trend to reduce IgE-associated diseases and prevented atopic eczema at 2 years Increased fecal lactobacilli and bifidobacteria	Kukkonen et al., 2007, 2008
L. rhamnosus GG	Intake by mothers at family-risk for 4 weeks before delivery and postnatally for 6 months	Risk reduction of atopic eczema for up to 7 years Increasing of TGF-β2 in mother's milk	Kalliomaki et al., 2007 Rautava et al., 2002
L. rhamnosus GG and *B. lactis* Bb2	Intake by pregnant women from the first trimester of pregnancy till the end of exclusive breast-feeding	Modest increase of TGF-β2 in colostrums Reduced allergen sensitization in infants	Huurre et al., 2008
L. rhamnosus GG	Intake by pregnant women for 36 weeks before delivery	No effect on fetal antigen-specific immune responses evaluated in cord blood cells	Boyle et al., 2008
L. rhamnosus GG	Intake by women at risk of atopic diseases from 4 to 6 weeks before delivery and postnatally for 6 months	No effect on incidence of atopic dermatitis	Kopp et al., 2008
Lactobacillus GG and *B. lactis* Bb12 plus dietary counselling	Intake by women from early till end of pregnancy	Increased placental concentrations of linoleic and dihomo-gamma-linolenic acids.	Kaplas et al., 2007
Dietary recommendations and *Lactobacillus* GG and *B. lactis*	Intake by women from first trimester of pregnancy onwards.	Highest and lowest intakes of specific nutrients associated with higher blood pressure in children at 6 months	Aaltonen et al., 2008
Lactobacillus GG and *B. lactis* Bb12 plus dietary counselling	Intake by women from first trimester of pregnancy onwards	Lowest blood glucose concentrations and highest glucose tolerance during pregnancy and over the 12 months postpartum	Laitinen et al., 2008

7.1. Influence of Maternal and Infant Probiotic Intake in Child Health

The use of probiotics during pregnancy is under consideration due to the positive effects of some strains on diverse clinical situations such as infections (vaginal, respiratory and gastrointestinal) and allergy, as well as on the physiological development of immune and metabolic functions. The number of human clinical trials intended to validate such probiotic an application is rapidly increasing, some of which are showing moderate effectiveness, improving child's health. The effectiveness of probiotics for preventing preterm labor and birth has been the objective of recent studies since the risk of this outcome in the presence of maternal infection is dramatically increased, reaching values of 30% to 50% (Othman et al., 2007). It has been suggested that specific probiotics could exert beneficial effects on such applications because of their ability to displace and inhibit pathogens and modulate immune responses by interfering with the inflammatory cascade that leads to preterm labor and delivery. So far, the two randomized controlled trials assessing the prevention of preterm birth in pregnant women and women planning pregnancy with the use of probiotics registered in 2006 have been reviewed (Othman et al., 2007). One study enrolled women after 34 weeks of pregnancy using oral fermented milk as probiotic, while the other study enrolled women diagnosed with bacterial vaginosis in early pregnancy that utilized commercially available yogurt vaginally. The results showed 81% reduction in the risk of genital infection with the use of probiotics. However, this was the only pre-specified clinical data available and there are, currently, insufficient data to assess impact on preterm birth and its complications (Othman et al., 2007). The prevention of AIDS and other infections in women and children by dietary intervention based on the probiotic concept has also been considered a possibility but still a distant reality (Reid & Devillard, 2004).

The use of probiotic bacteria during pregnancy could be a mean to modulate immune development in the fetus to reduce the risk of immune aberrancies and improve the host's defenses. In this context, the effects of the consumption of milk fermented with the strain *Lactobacillus casei* DN11401 by pregnant women during 6 weeks before delivery and during 6 weeks of lactation were determined (Ortiz-Andrellucchi et al., 2008). Mothers supplemented with the probiotic showed a significant increase in natural killer cells in peripheral blood samples and a non-significant increase in T and B lymphocytes. The pro-inflammatory cytokine TNF-α was decreased in maternal milk and breast-fed child of the mothers who consumed *L. casei* showed fewer gastrointestinal episodes. The safety and effects of a mixture of 4 probiotic bacterial strains (*Lactobacillus rhamnosus* GG and LC705, *Bifidobacterium breve* Bb99, and *Propionibacterium freudenreichii* ssp *shermanii*) with a prebiotic galacto-oligosaccharide has also been evaluated in pregnant women carrying high-risk children of allergic diseases and their infants. Pregnant women consumed a probiotic preparation or a placebo for 2 to 4 weeks before delivery and their infants received the same probiotics plus galacto-oligosaccharides for 6 months. No differences in growth, infant colic, morbidity or other adverse health effects between the two groups of children were found. Moreover, while 28 % of children in the placebo group had been prescribed antibiotics, only 23 % of children in the probiotic group had during the intervention. Respiratory infections also occurred less frequently in the synbiotic group (3.7 versus 4.2 mean infections) throughout the follow-up period (Kukkonen et al., 2008).

The administration of the probiotic *L. rhamnosus* GG to both pregnant mother and their babies has also been demonstrated to reduce the incidence of atopic eczema for up to 7 years in the Finish population (Kalliomaki et al., 2007). *L. rhamnosus* GG was given prenatally to mothers, who had at least one first-degree relative with atopic eczema, allergic rhinitis, or asthma, for 4 weeks before expected delivery and postnatally for 6 months to their children. *L. rhamnosus* GG was effective in prevention of early atopic disease in children at high risk as determined by considering chronic recurring atopic eczema as the primary endpoint. The administration of probiotics to the pregnant and lactating mother was shown to increase the amount of anti-inflammatory cytokine TGF-β2 in the mother's milk, thereby increasing its immunoprotective potential (Rautava et al., 2002). The infants most likely to benefit from maternal probiotic supplementation were those with an elevated cord blood IgE concentration (Rautava et al., 2002). In addition, Huurre et al. (2008b) evaluated the effects of dietary counselling and probiotic supplementation (*L. rhamnosus* GG and *B. lactis* Bb2) to pregnant women at risk of developing atopy on their children. Children of atopic mothers, specifically when breastfed exclusively over 2.5 months or 6 months, had a higher risk of sensitization at the age of 12 months but this risk could be reduced by the use of probiotics during pregnancy and lactation. The preventive effects were considered to be the result of a beneficial change in breast milk composition characterized by a modest increase in TGF-β2 concentration (Huurre et al., 2008b); however, this increase did not reach statistical significance and it was only detected in the colostrums while disappeared after 1 month. To progress on the knowledge of the mechanisms of action beyond the effects of *L. rhamnosus* GG intake on atopic eczema prevention, Boyle et al., (2008) investigated whether this probiotic influenced the fetal immune responses when administered to pregnant women for 36 week before delivery. The effects of stimulation of cord blood mononuclear cells from women who received the probiotic or placebo with heat-killed *L. rhamnosus* GG and ovalbumin were evaluated, without showing effects of the treatment on CD4(+) T cell proliferation, forkhead box P3 expression, dendritic cell phenotype or cytokine secretion. Therefore, *L. rhamnosus* GG supplementation to pregnant women failed to influence fetal antigen-specific immune responses and transplacental immune effects were excluded as the mechanisms of probiotic action (Boyle et al., 2008). The effects of a mixture of 4 probiotic bacterial strains (*L. rhamnosus* GG and LC705, *Bifidobacterium breve* Bb99, and *Propionibacterium freudenreichii* ssp *shermanii*) with galacto-oligosaccharides on allergic disease prevention were also evaluated in pregnant women carrying high-risk children. Pregnant women consumed a probiotic preparation or a placebo for 2 to 4 weeks before delivery and their infants received the same probiotics plus galacto-oligosaccharides or placebo for 6 months. Probiotic treatment compared with placebo showed no effect on the cumulative incidence of allergic diseases but tended to reduce IgE-associated (atopic) diseases and prevented atopic eczema at 2 years. In addition, lactobacilli and bifidobacteria more frequently colonized the intestine of supplemented infants, suggesting an inverse association between atopic diseases and gut colonization by probiotics (Kukkonen et al., 2007).

In spite of the aforementioned evidence, the value of probiotics for primary prevention of atopic diseases is still controversial. An additional clinical double-blind, placebo-controlled trial has been carried out to study the preventive effect of the same probiotic, *L. rhamnosus* GG, on the development of atopic dermatitis in Germany (Kopp et al., 2008). Pregnant women from families with 1 or more members with an atopic disease received either the probiotic or placebo from 4 to 6 weeks before expected delivery, followed by a postnatal period of 6 months. In this case, supplementation with *L. rhamnosus* GG during pregnancy and early infancy neither reduced the incidence of atopic dermatitis nor altered the severity of atopic dermatitis in affected children, but was associated with an increased rate of recurrent episodes of wheezing bronchitis at the age of 2 years. Therefore, the authors conclude that *L. rhamnosus* GG could not be generally recommended for primary prevention of atopic dermatitis (Kopp et al., 2008).

The metabolic effects of probiotic supplementation during the perinatal period also seem to be relevant to fetal programming and infant's development and metabolism. A pilot intervention program in which participants received either a combination of dietary counselling and probiotics (*Lactobacillus* GG and *B. lactis* Bb12), dietary counselling with placebo, or placebo alone from early pregnancy onwards showed significant effects of the intervention on placental lipids. The major differences in placental fatty acids were attributable to a higher concentration of n-3 polyunsaturated fatty acids in both intervention arms than in controls. Further, dietary counselling with probiotics resulted in higher concentrations of linoleic (18:2n-6) and dihomo-gamma-linolenic acids (20:3n-6) comparing with either dietary counselling with placebo or controls (Kaplas et al., 2007). The impact of maternal nutrition with probiotic supplementation during pregnancy on infant blood pressure has also been evaluated (Aaltonen et al., 2008). Pregnant women were randomized into 3 groups, the first submitted to a modified dietary intake according to current recommendations and probiotics (diet/probiotics), the second followed dietary recommendations and received placebo (diet/placebo), and the third received placebo (control/placebo). Although these results were not completely conclusive, the highest and lowest intakes of specific nutrients, such as carbohydrates and monounsaturated fatty acids compared with the middle ones were associated with higher blood pressure in children at the age 6 months, suggesting that dietary counselling can promote child health by programming blood pressure. The effects of probiotic supplementation together with dietary counselling on glucose metabolism in pregnant women were evaluated further leading to more conclusive results (Laitinen et al., 2008). The study included three subgroups of pregnant woman at the first trimester of pregnancy, the first group received nutrition counselling to modify dietary intake according to current recommendations (diet/placebo), the second group received nutrition counselling and probiotics (*L. rhamnosus* GG and *B. lactis* Bb12; diet/probiotics) and the third group received placebo without nutritional counselling (control/placebo). Blood glucose concentrations were the lowest in the diet/probiotics group during pregnancy and over the 12 months' postpartum period. Glucose tolerance was also better in the diet/probiotics group compared with the control/placebo group during the last trimester of pregnancy and over the 12-month postpartum period. Therefore, the study suggests that dietary counselling with probiotics can improved blood glucose control in a normoglycaemic population and, thus, may provide potential novel means for the prophylactic and therapeutic management of glucose disorders (Laitinen et al., 2008).

Conclusions and Future Perspectives

In the light of current scientific evidence, the potential of dietary interventions to improve the health of the mother and the infant is significant from conception onwards. Given the role of the intestinal microbiota in host immunity and metabolism, particularly at early developmental stages, dietary interventions based on probiotic and prebiotic administration could aid in health programming and disease prevention. To make it reality, further studies are needed to define the mechanisms by which intestinal bacterial may influence mothers physiology and the transmission routs of such effects to the offspring. The development of a larger number of clinical trials with different probiotic strains, in diverse physiological conditions and during well-established intervention time-frames could be of great help to extend the probiotic concept applications and reduce the burden of disease within the modern lifestyle context.

Acknowledgments

This work was supported by grants AGL2007-66126-C03-01/ALI and Consolider Fun-C-Food CSD2007-00063 from the Spanish Ministry of Science and Innovation and AP-124/09 from Consejería de Sanidad (Valencia, Spain).

References

Aaltonen, J., Ojala, T., Laitinen, K., Piirainen, T.J., Poussa, T.A. & Isolauri, E. (2008). Evidence of infant blood pressure programming by maternal nutrition during pregnancy: a prospective randomized controlled intervention study. *J. Pediatr.* 152, 79-84, 84.e1-2.

Adlerberth, I., Lindberg, E., Aberg, N., Hesselmar, B., Saalman, R., Strannegård, I.L. & Wold, A.E. (2006). Reduced enterobacterial and increased staphylococcal colonization of the infantile bowel: an effect of hygienic lifestyle? *Pediatr. Res.* 59, 96-101.

Ahrné, S., Lönnermark, E., Wold, A.E., Aberg, N., Hesselmar, B., Saalman, R., Strannegård, I.L., Molin, G. & Adlerberth, I. (2005). Lactobacilli in the intestinal microbiota of Swedish infants. *Microbes Infect.* 7, 256-62.

Ayabe, T., Satchell, D.P., Wilson, C.L., Parks, W.C., Selsted, M.E. & Ouellette, A.J. (2000). Secretion of microbicidal alpha-defensins by intestinal Paneth cells in response to bacteria. *Nat. Immunol.* 1, 113-8.

Bäckhed, F., Ding, H., Wang, T., Hooper, .LV., Koh, G.Y., Nagy, A., Semenkovich, C.F. & Gordon, J.I. (2004). The gut microbiota as an environmental factor that regulates fat storage. *Proc. Natl. Acad. Sci. U.S.A.* 101, 15718-23.

Bäckhed, F., Manchester, J.K., Semenkovich, C.F. & Gordon, J.I. (2007). Mechanisms underlying the resistance to diet-induced obesity in germ-free mice. *Proc. Natl. Acad. Sci. U.S.A.* 104, 979-84.

Bakker-Zierikzee, A.M., Tol, E.A., Kroes, H., Alles, M.S., Kok, F.J. & Bindels, J.G. (2006). Faecal SIgA secretion in infants fed on pre- or probiotic infant formula. *Pediatr. Allergy Immunol.* 17, 134-40.

Barker, D.J. (2007). The origins of the developmental origins theory. *J. Intern. Med.* 261, 412-7.

Berg, R.D. (1996). The indigenous gastrointestinal microflora. Trends Microbiol. 4, 430–435.

Bertino, E., Bisson, C., Martano, C., Coscia, A., Fabris, C., Monti, G., Testa, T. & Conti, A. (2006). Relationship between maternal- and fetal-specific IgE. *Pediatr. Allergy Immunol.* 17, 484-8.

Biasucci, G., Benenati, B., Morelli, L., Bessi, E. & Boehm, G. (2008). Cesarean delivery may affect the early biodiversity of intestinal bacteria. *J. Nutr.* 138,1796S-1800S.

Björkstén, B. (2006). The gut microbiota: a complex ecosystem. *Clin. Experimental Allergy.* 36,1215-1217.

Blümer, N., Sel, S., Virna, S., Patrascan, C.C., Zimmermann, S., Herz, U., Renz, H. & Garn, H. (2007). Perinatal maternal application of *Lactobacillus rhamnosus* GG suppresses allergic airway inflammation in mouse offspring. *Clin. Exp. Allergy.* 37, 348-57.

Boyle, R.J., Mah, L.J., Chen, A., Kivivuori, S., Robins-Browne, R.M. & Tang, M.L. (2008). Effects of *Lactobacillus* GG treatment during pregnancy on the development of fetal antigen-specific immune responses. *Clin. Exp. Allergy.* 38, 1882-90.

Caballero-Franco, C., Keller, K., De Simone, C. & Chadee, K. (2007). The VSL#3 probiotic formula induces mucin gene expression and secretion in colonic epithelial cells. *Am. J. Physiol. Gastrointest. Liver Physiol.* 292, 315-22.

Calder, P.C., Krauss-Etschmann, S., de Jong, E.C., Dupont, C., Frick, J.S., Frokiaer, H., Heinrich, J., Garn, H., Koletzko, S., Lack, G., Mattelio, G.,

Renz, H., Sangild, P.T., Schrezenmeir, J., Stulnig, T.M., Thymann, T., Wold, A.E. & Koletzko, B. (2006). Early nutrition and immunity - progress and perspectives. *Br. J. Nutr.* 96, 774-90.

Cash, H.L., Whitham, C.V., Behrendt ,C.L.& Hooper, L.V. (2006). Symbiotic bacteria direct expression of an intestinal bactericidal lectin. *Science.* 313,1126-30.

Chen, J., Cai, W. & Feng, Y. (2007). Development of intestinal bifidobacteria and lactobacilli in breast-fed neonates. *Clin. Nutr.* 26, 559-66.

Church, M.W., Jen, K.L., Jackson, D.A., Adams, B.R. & Hotra, J.W. (2009). Abnormal neurological responses in young adult offspring caused by excess omega-3 fatty acid (fish oil) consumption by the mother during pregnancy and lactation. *Neurotoxicol. Teratol.* 31, 26-33.

Ege, M.J., Herzum, I., Büchele, G., Krauss-Etschmann, S., Lauener, R.P., Bitter, S., Roponen, M., Remes, S., Vuitton, D.A., Riedler, J. Brunekreef, B., Dalphin, J.C., Braun-Fahrländer, C., Pekkanen, J., Renz, H. von Mutius, E. & PASTURE Study Group. (2008) Specific IgE to allergens in cord blood is associated with maternal immunity to Toxoplasma gondii and rubella virus. *Allergy.* 63, 1505-11.

Fåk, F,, Ahrné, S., Molin, G., Jeppsson, B. & Weström, B. (2008). Maternal consumption of *Lactobacillus plantarum* 299v affects gastrointestinal growth and function in the suckling rat. *Br. J. Nutr.* 100, 332-8.

FAO/WHO working group (2002). Guidelines for the Evaluation of Probiotics in Food. *ftp://ftp. fao. org/es/esn/food/wgreport2. pdf.*

Favier, C.F., de Vos, W.M. & Akkermans, A.D. (2003). Development of bacterial and bifidobacterial communities in feces of newborn babies. *Anaerobe.* 9, 219-29.

Freitas, M., Axelsson, L.G., Cayuela, C., Midtvedt, T. & Truenan, G. (2005). Indigenous microbes and their soluble factors differentially modulate intestinal glycosylation steps in vivo. Use of a "lectin assay" to survey in vivo glycosylation changes. *Histochem. Cell Biol.* 124, 423-33.

Gill, S.R., Pop, M., Deboy, R.T., Eckburg, P.B., Turnbaugh, P.J., Samuel, B.S., Gordon, J.I., Relman, D.A., Fraser-Liggett, C.M. & Nelson, K.E. (2006). Metagenomic analysis of the human distal gut microbiome. *Science.* 312, 1355-9.

González, R., Klaassens, E.S., Marinen, E., de Vos, W.M. & Vaughan, E.E. (2008). Differential transcriptional response of Bifidobacterium longum to human milk,formula milk, and galactooligosaccharide. *Appl. Environ. Microbiol.* 74, 4686-94.

Grangeot-Keros, L., Pillot, J., Daffos, F. & Forestier, F. (1988). Prenatal and postnatal production of IgM and IgA antibodies to rubella virus studied by antibody capture immunoassay. *J. Infect. Dis.* 158, 138-43.

Grönlund, M.M., Arvilommi, H., Kero, P., Lehtonen, O.P. & Isolauri, E. (2000). Importance of intestinal colonisation in the maturation of humoral immunity in early infancy: a prospective follow up study of healthy infants aged 0-6 months. *Arch. Dis. Child Fetal Neonatal Ed.* 83, F186-92.

Grönlund, M.-M., M. Gueimonde, K. Laitinen, G. Kociubinski, T. Grönroos, S. Salminen, & E. Isolauri. (2007). Maternal breast-milk and intestinal bifidobacteria guide the compositional development of the *Bifidobacterium* microbiota in infants at risk of allergic disease. *Clin. Exp. Allergy.* 37, 1764-1772.

Gueimonde, M., Sakata, S., Kalliomäki, M., Isolauri, E., Benno, Y. & Salminen, S. (2006). Effect of maternal consumption of *Lactobacillus* GG on transfer and establishment of fecal bifidobacterial microbiota in neonates. *J. Pediatr. Gastroenterol. Nutr.* 42, 166-70.

Gueimonde M, Laitinen K, Salminen S, Isolauri E. Breast milk: a source of bifidobacteria for infant gut development and maturation? *Neonatology.* 2007;92(1):64-6.

Haarman, M. & Knol, J. (2005). Quantitative real-time PCR assays to identify and quantify fecal *Bifidobacterium* species in infants receiving a prebiotic infant formula. *Appl. Environ. Microbiol.* 71, 2318-24.

Herrera, E. (2002). Implications of dietary fatty acids during pregnancy on placental, fetal and postnatal development--a review. *Placenta.* 23, Suppl A:S9-19.

Hooper, L.V., Wong, M.H., Thelin, A., Hansson, L., Falk, P.G. & Gordon, J.I. (2001). Molecular analysis of commensal host-microbial relationships in the intestine. *Science.* 291, 881-4.

Hooper, L.V., Midtvedt, T. & Gordon, J.I. (2002). How host-microbial interactions shape the nutrient environment of the mammalian intestine. *Annu. Rev. Nutr.* 22, 283-307.

Hooper, L.V., Stappenbeck, T.S., Hong, C.V. & Gordon, J.I.(2003). Angiogenins: a new class of microbicidal proteins involved in innate immunity. *Nat. Immunol.* 4, 269-73.

Hrncir, T., Stepankova, R., Kozakova, H., Hudcovic, T. & Tlaskalova-Hogenova, H. (2008). Gut microbiota and lipopolysaccharide content of the diet influence development of regulatory T cells: studies in germ-free mice. *BMC Immunol.* 6,9:65.

Huurre, A., Kalliomäki, M., Rautava, S., Rinne, M., Salminen, S. & Isolauri, E. (2008a). Mode of delivery - effects on gut microbiota and humoral immunity. *Neonatology.* 93, 236-40.

Huurre, A., Laitinen, K., Rautava, S., Korkeamäki, M. & Isolauri E. (2008b). Impact of maternal atopy and probiotic supplementation during pregnancy on infant sensitization: a double-blind placebo-controlled study. *Clin. Exp. Allergy.* 38, 1342-8.

Inoue, R., Otsuka, M. & Ushida, K.(2005). Development of intestinal microbiota in mice and its possible interaction with the evolution of luminal IgA in the intestine. *Exp. Anim.* 54, 437-45.

Kalliomaki, M., Salminen, S., Poussa, T. & Isolauri, E. (2007). Probiotics during the first 7 years of life: a cumulative risk reduction of eczema in a randomized, placebo-controlled trial. *J. Allergy Clin. Immunol.* 119, 1019-21.

Kaplas, N., Isolauri, E., Lampi, A.M., Ojala, T. & Laitinen, K. (2007). Dietary counseling and probiotic supplementation during pregnancy modif. placental phospholipid fatty acids. *Lipids.* 42, 865-70.

Kelly, D., Campbell, J.I., King, T.P., Grant, G., Jansson, E.A., Coutts, A.G., Pettersson ,S. & Conway, S. (2004). Commensal anaerobic gut bacteria attenuate inflammation by regulating nuclear-cytoplasmic shuttling of PPAR-gamma and RelA. *Nat. Immunol.* 5, 104-12.

Kelly, G. (2008). Inulin-type prebiotics - a review: part 1. *Altern. Med. Rev.* 13, 316-330.

Kopp, M.V., Goldstein, M., Dietschek, A., Sofke, J., Heinzmann, A. & Urbanek, R. (2008). *Lactobacillus* GG has in vitro effects on enhanced interleukin-10 and interferon-gamma release of mononuclear cells but no in vivo effects in supplemented mothers and their neonates. *Clin. Exp. Allergy.* 38, 602-10.

Kramer, D.R. & Cebra, J.J. (1995). Early appearance of "natural" mucosal IgA responses and germinal centers in suckling mice developing in the absence of maternal antibodies. *J. Immunol.* 154, 2051-62.

Kukkonen, K., Savilahti, E., Haahtela, T., Juntunen-Backman, K., Korpela, R., Poussa, T., Tuure, T. & Kuitunen, M. (2007). Probiotics and prebiotic galacto-oligosaccharides in the prevention of allergic diseases: a randomized, double-blind, placebo-controlled trial. *J. Allergy Clin. Immunol.* 119, 192-8.

Kukkonen, K., Savilahti, E., Haahtela, T., Juntunen-Backman, K., Korpela, R., Poussa, T., Tuure, T. & Kuitunen, M. (2008). Long-term safety and impact on infection rates of postnatal probiotic and prebiotic (synbiotic) treatment: randomized, double-blind, placebo-controlled trial. *Pediatrics*. 122, 8-12.

Laitinen, K., Poussa, T., Isolauri, E. & the Nutrition, Allergy, Mucosal Immunology and Intestinal Microbiota Group. (2008). Probiotics and dietary counselling contribute to glucose regulation during and after pregnancy: a randomised controlled trial. *Br. J. Nutr.* 19, 1-9.

Lamb, M.M., Myers, M.A., Barriga, K., Zimmet, P.Z., Rewers, M. & Norris, J.M. (2008). Maternal diet during pregnancy and islet autoimmunity in offspring. *Pediatr. Diabetes.* 9, 135-41.

Lee, J., Rachmilewitz, D. & Raz, E. (2006). Homeostatic effects of TLR9 signaling in experimental colitis. *Ann. N. Y. Acad. Sci.* 1072, 351-5.

Ley, R.E., Lozupone, C.A., Hamady, M., Knight, R. & Gordon, J.I. (2008). Worlds within worlds: evolution of the vertebrate gut microbiota. *Nat. Rev. Microbiol.* 6, 776-88.

Lindberg, E., Adlerberth, I., Hesselmar, B., Saalman, R., Strannegård, I.L., Aberg, N. & Wold A.E. (2004). High rate of transfer of *Staphylococcus aureus* from parental skin to infant gut flora. *J. Clin. Microbiol.* 42, 530-4.

LoCascio, R.G., Ninonuevo, M.R., Freeman, S.L., Sela, D.A., Grimm, R., Lebrilla, C.B., Mills, D.A. & German, J.B. (2007). Glycoprofiling of bifidobacterial consumption of human milk oligosaccharides demonstrates strain specific, preferential consumption of small chain glycans secreted in early human lactation. *J. Agric Food Chem.* 55, 8914-9.

Lodinova-Zadnikova, R., Cukrowska, B. & Tlaskalova-Hogenova, H. (2003). Oral administration of probiotic *Escherichia coli* after birth reduces frequency of allergies and repeated infections later in life (after 10 and 20 years). *Int. Arch. Allergy Immunol.*.131, 209-11.

Lussana, F., Painter, R.C., Ocke, M.C., Buller, H.R., Bossuyt, P.M. & Roseboom, T.J. (2008). Prenatal exposure to the Dutch famine is associated with a preference for fatty foods and a more atherogenic lipid profile. *Am. J. Clin. Nutr.* 88, 1648-52.

Lutgendorff, F., Akkermans, L.M. & Söderholm, J.D. (2008). The role of microbiota and probiotics in stress-induced gastro-intestinal damage. *Curr. Mol. Med.* 8, 282-98.

Mack, D.R., Ahrne, S., Hyde, L., Wei, S. & Hollingsworth, M.A. (2003). Extracellular MUC3 mucin secretion follows adherence of *Lactobacillus* strains to intestinal epithelial cells in vitro. *Gut.* 52, 827-33.

Mackie, R.I., Sghir, A. & Gaskins, H.R. (1999). Developmental microbial ecology of the neonatal gastrointestinal tract. *Am. J. Clin. Nutr.* 69, 1035S-1045S.

Martín, R., Jiménez, E., Heilig, H., Fernández, L., Marín, M.L., Zoetendal, E.G. & Rodríguez J.M. (2008). Isolation of bifidobacteria from breast milk and assessment of the bifidobacterial population by PCR-DGGE and qRTi-PCR. *Appl. Environ. Microbiol.* 2008 Dec 16. [Epub ahead of print]

McCracken, V.J. & Lorenz, R.G. (2001). The gastrointestinal ecosystem: a precarious alliance among epithelium, immunity and microbiota. *Cell Microbiol.* 3, 1–11.

McCurdy, C.E., Bishop, J.M., Williams, S.M., Grayson, B.E., Smith, M.S., Friedman, J.E. & Grove, K.L. (2009). Maternal high-fat diet triggers lipotoxicity in the fetal livers of nonhuman primates. *J. Clin. Invest.* Jan 19. pii: 32661. doi: 10.1172/JCI32661.

McDonagh, S., Maidji, E., Ma, W. Chang, H.T., Fisher, S. & Pereira, L. (2004). Viral and bacterial pathogens at the maternal-fetal interface. *Infect. Dis.* 190, 826-34.

Mevissen-Verhage, E.A., Marcelis, J.H., de Vos, M.N., Harmsen-van Amerongen, W.C. & Verhoef, J. (1987). *Bifidobacterium, Bacteroides,* and *Clostridium* spp. in fecal samples from breast-fed and bottle-fed infants with and without iron supplement. *J. Clin. Microbiol.* 25, 285-9.

Mitsuoka, T. & Kaneuchi, C. (1977). Ecology of the bifidobacteria. *Am. J. Clin. Nutr.* 30, 1799-810.

Munakata, K., Yamamoto, M., Anjiki, N., Nishiyama, M., Imamura, S., Iizuka, S., Takashima, K., Ishige, A., Hioki, K., Ohnishi, Y. & Watanabe K. (2008). Importance of the interferon-alpha system in murine large intestine indicated by microarray analysis of commensal bacteria-induced immunological changes. *BMC Genomics.* 26;9:192.

Neish, A.S., Gewirtz, A.T., Zeng, H., Young, A.N., Hobert, M.E., Karmali, V., Rao, A.S. & Madara, J.L. (2000). Prokaryotic regulation of epithelial responses by inhibition of IkappaB-alpha ubiquitination. *Science.* 289, 1560-3.

Ortiz-Andrellucchi, A., Sánchez-Villegas, A., Rodríguez-Gallego, C., Lemes, A., Molero, Soria, A., Peña-Quintana, L., Santana, M., Ramírez, O., García, J., Cabrera, F., Cobo, J., Serra-Majem, L. (2008). Immunomodulatory effects of the intake of fermented milk with *Lactobacillus casei* DN114001 in lactating mothers and their children. *Br. J. Nutr.* 100, 834-45.

Othman, M., Neilson, J.P. & Alfirevic, Z. (2007). Probiotics for preventing preterm labour. *Cochrane Database Syst. Rev.* 24, (1):CD005941.

Otte, J.M., Cario, E. & Podolsky, D.K. (2004). Mechanisms of cross hyporesponsiveness to Toll-like receptor bacterial ligands in intestinal epithelial cells. *Gastroenterology.* 126, 1054-70.

Palmer, C., Bik, E.M., Digiulio, D.B., Relman, D.A. & Brown, P.O. (2007). Development of the Human Infant Intestinal Microbiota. *PLoS Biol.* 26; 5(7):e177.

Penders, J., Thijs, C., Vink, C., Stelma, F.F., Snijders, B., Kummeling, I., van den Brandt, P.A. & Stobberingh, E.E. (2006). Factors influencing the composition of the intestinal microbiota in early infancy. *Pediatrics.* 118, 511-21.

Polte, T., Hennig, C. & Hansen, G. (2008). Allergy prevention starts before conception: maternofetal transfer of tolerance protects against the development of asthma. *J. Allergy Clin. Immunol.* 122, 1022-1030.e5.

Rautava, S., Kalliomaki, M. & Isolauri, E. (2002). Probiotics during pregnancy and breast-feeding might confer immunomodulatory protection against atopic disease in the infant. *J. Allergy Clin. Immunol.* 109, 119-21.

Reid, G. & Devillard, E. (2004). Probiotics for mother and child. *J. Clin. Gastroenterol.* 38, (6 Suppl) S94-101.

Roberfroid, M. (2007). Prebiotics: the concept revisited. *J. Nutr.* 137, 830-7.

Salminen, S. & Isolauri, E. (2006). Intestinal colonization, microbiota, and probiotics. *J. Pediatr.* 149, S115-S120.

Sanz, Y., Nadal, I. & Sánchez, E. (2007a). Probiotics as drugs against human gastrointestinal infections. *Recent Pat. Antiinfect. Drug Discov.* 2, 148-56.

Sanz, Y. (2007b). Ecological and functional implications of the acid-adaptation ability of *Bifidobacterium*: a way of selecting improved probiotic strains. *Int. Dairy J.* 17, 1284-1289.

Sanz, Y., Sánchez, E., De Palma, G., Medina, M., Marcos, A. & Nova, E. (2008a). Indigenous gut microbiota, probiotics, and coeliac disease. In: *Child Nutrition & Physiology.* Linda T. Overton & M R. Ewente, Eds. Nova Science Publishers, Inc, NY, USA. pp. 210-224.

Sanz, Y., Santacruz, A. & De Palma G. (2008b). Insights into the roles of gut microbes in obesity. The Human Microbiome and Infectious Diseases: Beyond Koch. *Interdisciplinary Perspectives on Infectious Diseases.* doi: 10.1155/2008/829101.

Satokari, R., Grönroos, T., Laitinen, K., Salminen, S. & Isolauri, E. (2008). *Bifidobacterium* and *Lactobacillus* DNA in the human placenta. *Lett. Appl. Microbiol.* Oct 17. [Epub ahead of print]

Sawada, J., Morita, H., Tanaka, A., Salminen, S., He, F. & Matsuda, H. (2007). Ingestion of heat-treated *Lactobacillus rhamnosus* GG prevents development of atopic dermatitis in NC/Nga mice. *Clin. Exp. Allergy.* 37, 296-303.

Scholtens, P.A., Alles, M.S., Bindels, J.G., van der Linde, E.G., Tolboom, J.J. & Knol, J. (2006). Bifidogenic effects of solid weaning foods with added prebiotic oligosaccharides: a randomised controlled clinical trial. *J. Pediatr. Gastroenterol. Nutr.* 42, 553-9.

Schultz, M,, Göttl, C., Young, R.J., Iwen, P. & Vanderhoof, J.A. (2004). Administration of oral probiotic bacteria to pregnant women causes temporary infantile colonization. *J. Pediatr. Gastroenterol. Nutr.* 38, 293-7.

Schwiertz, A., Gruhl, B., Lobnitz, M., Michel, P., Radke, M. & Blaut, M. (2003). Development of the intestinal bacterial composition in hospitalized preterm infants in comparison with breast-fed, full-term infants. *Pediatr. Res.* 54, 393–9.

Sela, D.A., Chapman, J., Adeuya, A., Kim, J.H., Chen, F., Whitehead, T.R,, Lapidus, A., Rokhsar, D.S., Lebrilla, C.B., German, J.B., Price, N.P., Richardson, P.M. & Mills, D.A. (2008). The genome sequence of *Bifidobacterium longum* subsp. *infantis* reveals adaptations for milk utilization within the infant microbiome. *Proc. Natl. Acad. Sci. U.S.A.* 105, 18964-9.

Siggers, R.H., Siggers, J., Boye, M. Thymann, T., Mølbak, L., Leser, T., Jensen, B.B. & Sangild, P.T. (2008). Early administration of probiotics alters bacterial colonization and limits diet-induced gut dysfunction and severity of necrotizing enterocolitis in preterm pigs. *J. Nutr.* 138, 1437-44.

Solano-Aguilar, G., Dawson, H., Restrepo, M., Andrews, K,. Vinyard, B. & Urban, J.F. Jr. (2008). Detection of *Bifidobacterium animalis* subsp. *lactis* (Bb12) in the intestine after feeding of sows and their piglets. *Appl. Environ. Microbiol.* 74, 6338-47.

Stappenbeck, T.S., Hooper, L.V. & Gordon, J.I. (2002). Developmental regulation of intestinal angiogenesis by indigenous microbes via Paneth cells. *Proc. Natl. Acad. Sci. U.S.A.* 99, 15451-5.

Stewart, J.A., Chadwick, V.S. & Murray, A. (2005). Investigations into the influence of host genetics on the predominant eubacteria in the faecal microflora of children. *J. Med. Microbiol.* 54, 1239-42.

Strachan, D.P. (1989). Hay fever, hygiene, and household size. *BMJ.* 299, 259-60.

Vaishnava, S., Behrendt, C.L., Ismail, A.S., Eckmann, L. & Hooper, L.V. (2008). Paneth cells directly sense gut commensals and maintain homeostasis at the intestinal host-microbial interface. *Proc. Natl. Acad. Sci. U.S.A.* 105, 20858-63.

Watanabe, T., Asano, N., Murray, P.J., Ozato, K., Tailor, P., Fuss, I.J., Kitani, A. & Strober, W. (2008). Muramyl dipeptide activation of nucleotide-binding oligomerization domain 2 protects mice from experimental colitis. *J. Clin. Invest.* 118, 545-59.

Westerbeek, E.A., van den Berg, A., Lafeber, H.N., Knol, J., Fetter, W.P. & van Elburg, R.M. (2006). The intestinal bacterial colonisation in preterm infants: a review of the literature. *Clin. Nutr.* 25, 361-8.

Winkler, P., Ghadimi, D., Schrezenmeir, J. & Kraehenbuhl, J.P. (2007). Molecular and cellular basis of microflora-host interactions. *J. Nutr.* 137(3 Suppl 2), 756S-72S.

Yajnik, C. (2006). Nutritional control of fetal growth. *Nutr. Rev.* 64 5 Pt 2),S50-1; S72-91.

Yates, Z., Tarling, E.J., Langley-Evans, S.C. & Salter AM. (2008). Maternal undernutrition programmes atherosclerosis in the ApoE*3-Leiden mouse. *Br. J. Nutr.* 10,1-10.

Zoetendal, E.G., Akkermans, A.D. & De Vos, W.M. (1998). Temperature gradient gel electrophoresis analysis of 16S rRNA from human fecal samples reveals stable and host-specific communities of active bacteria. *Appl. Environ. Microbiol.* 64, 3854-9.

Zoetendal, E.G., Akkermans, A.D.L., Akkermans-van Vliet, W.M. & De Vos, W.M. (2001). The host genotype affects the bacterial community in the human gastrointestinal tract. *Microb. Ecol. Health Dis.* 13, 129-34.

In: Pregnancy and Infants
Editor: Tsisana Shartava

ISBN 978-1-61209-132-7
© 2011 Nova Science Publishers, Inc.

Chapter 5

CLINICAL STAFF PERCEPTIONS OF THE TREATMENT OF PROCEDURAL PAIN IN NEONATES: EXPLORING A CHANGE PROCESS

Randi Dovland Andersen[*1], *Alf Meberg*[2], *Lars Wallin*[3,4] *and Leena Jylli*[3,5]

[1]Department of Pediatrics, Telemark Hospital, Skien, Norway
[2]Department of Pediatrics, Vestfold Hospital, Tonsberg, Norway
[3]Department of Neurobiology, Care Sciences and Society, Division of Nursing, Karolinska Institutet, Stockholm, Sweden
[4]Clinical Research Utilization (CRU), Karolinska University Hospital, Stockholm, Sweden
[5]Acute Pain Treatment Service, Astrid Lindgren Children's Hospital, Karolinska University Hospital, Stockholm, Sweden

---

[*] Corresponding author: Randi Dovland Andersen, RN. Pediatric Department. Telemark hospital. Ulefossveien. N-3710 Skien. Norway. E-mail: anrd@sthf.no.

ABSTRACT

Background: The gap between scientific knowledge and clinical practice is a major challenge in neonatal pain management. The aim of this study was to describe the clinicians' perceptions concerning the treatment of procedural pain in neonates, before and after the implementation of new pain-management strategies.

Methods: A multifaceted approach to changing practice was evaluated among nurses and physicians in two 16 beds neonatal intensive care units in southern Norway. The intervention included the establishment of an organizational framework for the change process, the development and implementation of evidence-based guidelines and procedures, education and local facilitators that assisted clinicians in changing their practice. Data were collected before and after the intervention, using a questionnaire. Ten commonly performed procedures were assessed. The response rates were 79% and 73%, respectively.

Results: Clinicians' answers indicated a slight increase in the actual use of pharmacological agents. Only the nurses reported changes in their views of procedure painfulness, the actual use of comfort measures, and the perceived optimal treatment for procedural pain. The intervention did not result in more concordant perceptions of physicians and nurses, neither in comprehensive changes in the treatment of procedural pain in neonates. Despite the performance of a multifaceted intervention to support evidence-based practice, the overall results point clearly to the difficulties in applying evidence to practice.

Keywords: Neonatal pain management, perceptions, survey, implementation of change, knowledge translation, clinical guidelines.

INTRODUCTION

One of the major challenges in neonatal pain management is the persistent gap between scientific knowledge and clinical practice [1]. The dissemination of scientific knowledge into clinical practice takes time, but a lack of knowledge alone cannot explain the discrepancy between available evidence and practice. Studies have shown that although knowledge can be well developed and appropriate, clinical practice does not change accordingly [2, 3]. Therefore, it is necessary to explore how scientific knowledge about neonatal pain management can be implemented in clinical practice.

Pain in neonates

All neonates have the functional capacity to experience pain at birth, but their nervous systems are still immature. This causes a prolonged and enhanced pain experience compared with that of older children or adults and makes neonates more vulnerable to the deleterious effects of pain [4].

In the past, the belief that neonates are unable to feel or respond to pain were common. The scientific work of Anand [5] and changes in public opinion caused by parental lobbying contributed to a new perspective on infant pain in the late 1980s [6]. The continuous advances in perinatal care have resulted in an extensive use of invasive and often painful procedures [7]. Assessing pain in neonates remains a great challenge because this group of patients cannot express their pain verbally [8]. Structured pain-assessment measures are underutilized in NICUs [9-11]. Instead, clinicians observe infant behavior and physiological parameters, identify signs of pain, and use these observations and their knowledge to determine whether infants are in pain and whether they require pain treatment [12].

Efficient pain management is based on a combination of different approaches, and include shielding the neonate from light, sounds, and unnecessary handling or procedures, choosing the least painful procedure, combining both different comfort measures as well as comfort measures and analgesics for optimal pain relief [13]. Blood sampling is one of the most common procedures performed in neonates. The associated pain can be lessened by performing blood sampling with venous punctures instead of the more painful heel sticks [14]. Despite the scientific advances over the past decades, pain in neonates is still poorly treated. Several studies have demonstrated a failure to treat pain in neonates efficiently, even for the most painful procedures [2, 7, 9-11, 15]. The need to narrow the knowledge–practice gap is obvious; unrelieved pain results in unnecessary suffering and early pain may have a substantial effect on later cognitive, social, and emotional functioning [16].

Implementation Research

Implementation research, or knowledge translation (i.e., research on how to put evidence to practice), is an emerging field in health care science [17]. The use of research has been on the health care agenda for a long time but has received greater prominence only in the last two decades. Neonatal pain management is a clinical area with great potential for improvement if available knowledge more often is put into action. Several systematic reviews have been published on interventions intended to change practitioners' behavior. At present, however, there is no knowledge base to draw on to develop recommendations on which intervention to use in a given setting [18].

The influence of individual factors has been investigated extensively [19], and it appears that the difficulties in implementing evidence might be explained largely in terms of contextual influences. Context is a vide concept, one important dimension being the social dimension. Social learning theory explains how the social setting can influence individuals' behavior and act as an imperative on individual behavioral change. The social setting both defines a frame of reference for behavior, and is a source of knowledge and information. Learning occurs by observation or imitation of what constitutes acceptable behavior in the group. The experience of rewards or unfavorable results plays an important role in shaping behavior, together with cognitive processes [20].

Rationale of This Study

In 2002, McGrath and Unruh [6] described change as a social process, stating that social influence is a necessary prerequisite for change, together with scientific and technical knowledge. When this study was planned, little systematic work had been done on the implementation of change in the field of neonatal pain management, therefore the intervention were based on the ideas of McGrath and Unruh and social learning theory [20].

It was assumed that the change of pain management practice had the following premises: Knowledge is a necessary but not sufficient prerequisite for change and must be disseminated and made available to all members of the group. Clinical practice is influenced by both individual and social/contextual factors, and a strategy to change clinical practice must target both. Multiprofessional interventions are necessary; no health professional can adequately manage pain alone.

The intervention was conducted in two NICUs in southern Norway. The clinicians' perceptions of the treatment of procedural pain in neonates prior to the intervention have been reported previously [2] and findings indicated that clinical practice was not in accordance with available guidelines [21, 22].

The aim of this paper is to describe the clinicians' perceptions concerning the treatment of procedural pain in neonates, before and after the implementation of new pain management strategies. We hypothesized that the respondents' answers would indicate an increase in the use of both pharmacological agents and comfort measures as well as greater agreement between the perceptions of nurses and physicians.

METHODS

Subjects and Setting

Physicians and nurses working in two 16 beds NICUs in southern Norway were eligible for participation in the questionnaire study $(N = 92)$. Approximately 2/3 of the respondents (n=73) answered the questionnaire at both time points. Table I shows the characteristics of the sample.

Table 1. Demographic characteristics of the sample

	2003	2005	P value
Number of respondents and percentage of the total population $(N = 92)$	73 (79)	67 (73)	
Hospital I, n (%)	38 (52)	33 (49)	0.866
Hospital II, n (%)	35 (48)	34 (51)	0.866
Physicians, n (%)	20 (27)	17 (25)	0.849
Nurses, n (%)	53 (73)	50 (75)	0.849
Senior pediatricians (n) and % of total physicians	11 (55)	8 (47)	0.746
Specialist nurses (n) and % of total nurses	13 (25)	16 (32)	0.511
Nurses who participated in the external competence program (n) and % of total nurses	21 (40)	39 (78)	0.001*
Age (mean ± SD) in years	39.6 ± 8.2	42.1 ± 10.4	0.116
Female, n (%)	59 (81)	52 (78)	0.680
Experience > 12 years, n (%)	29 (40)	30 (45)	0.699

Instrument

The data collection was based on a questionnaire, developed by Porter and colleagues [15], which consisted of a series of questions on pain and pain management with reference to 12 procedures frequently performed in neonates. In our study, 10 of the procedures were included (Table II). Circumcision and arterial or venous cutdown were excluded because these procedures were not performed in the units being studied. The responses were in a Likert-scale format, and the participants were asked to grade the painfulness of the 10 procedures, the frequencies of the actual use of pharmacological agents and comfort measures, and the optimal use of such measures (Table II).

Definitions

- Procedure: A therapeutic or diagnostic intervention carried out in neonates by health personnel
- Pharmacological agents: Paracetamol (acetaminophen), opioids, and/or local anesthetics.
- Comfort measures: Containment and support during a procedure, reduction of stimuli, nonnutritive sucking, sweet-tasting solutions, warming of the heel before a heel stick, and others.
- Procedure painfulness: The painfulness of each procedure, rated by the respondent on a five-item ordinal scale from "not painful" to "very painful".
- Actual use of pharmacological agents/comfort measures: The respondents' scoring on how often each procedure *was* performed accompanied with pharmacological agents/comfort measures, on a five-item ordinal scale from "never" to "always".
- Optimal use of pharmacological agents/comfort measures: The respondents' scoring on how often each procedure *should be* performed accompanied with pharmacological agents/comfort measures, on a five-item ordinal scale from "never" to "always".

Table II. Infant pain questionnaire

The following procedures were evaluated.	
INTU	Endotracheal intubation
TUBE	Insertion of chest tube
GAV	Insertion of gavage tube
SUCT	Tracheal suctioning
LP	Lumbar puncture
SHOT	Intramuscular injection
UAC	Insertion of umbilical catheter
PIV	Insertion of peripheral intravenous line
STK	Heel stick
RAC	Insertion of radial or tibial arterial catheter

Questions

1) Rate the painfulness of each procedure.

2) Rate how often you believe each procedure is performed using pharmacological agents (e.g., paracetamol, opioids, and/or local anesthetics).

3) Rate how often you believe each procedure is performed using comfort measures (e.g., containment and support during the procedure, reduction of stimuli, nonnutritive sucking, sweet-tasting solutions, warming of the heel before a heel stick, or others).

4) Rate how often you believe each procedure should be performed using pharmacological agents.

5) Rate how often you believe each procedure should be performed using comfort measures.

Questions were answered by the clinical staff according to the following scales.

Question 1	*Questions 2–5*
0 = not painful	0 = never
1 = somewhat painful	1 = rarely
2 = moderately painful	2 = often
3 = quite painful	3 = usually
4 = very painful	4 = always

Procedures and Intervention Program

Ethical approval for the study was obtained from the Regional Ethics Committee in southern Norway. A multifaceted intervention was designed, based on the theoretical underpinnings described above. The intervention included the establishment of an organizational framework for the change process, the development and implementation of evidence-based guidelines and procedures for blood collection, education and local facilitators that assisted clinicians in changing their practice. The intervention was carried out in three different phases.

1. Planning

A study protocol was drafted, and locally adapted, evidence-based guidelines were developed. The guidelines contained information on pain in neonates, pain assessment, and pain management with pharmacological agents and comfort measures, and were based on international [21] and Swedish national guidelines [22]. The intervention was organized as a project, but with close ties to the management at both pediatric departments. A multiprofessional project group (physician, nurse, and nurse assistant) was established at each hospital. Their task was to act as facilitators and assist in the implementation of the guidelines and the new procedure for blood collection at their own unit. Collaboration between the two project groups were planned. The management of both pediatric departments supported the project and provided initial funding. In addition to the establishment of close connections to the organizational leadership at both departments, the senior neonatologists at both NICUs were included in the drafting of the project and approved the medical content of the intervention.

2. Implementation

The implementation phase was initiated by one-day neonatal pain-management seminars, two at each unit. The education was based on the new guidelines, including the development, anatomy, and physiology of the pain system, the consequences of pain, pain assessment, pharmacological treatments, and environmental and behavioral pain-management strategies. Almost all the nurses and some of the physicians attended the seminars. To compensate for the lack of physician attendance, they were provided information in separate educational sessions. The local guidelines were made available in both units after the completion of all pain-management seminars and educational sessions.

The project manager and the members of the project groups performed their daily work in the units, acted as role models regarding pain management, and supported colleagues when various pain management issues arose. This support was most often carried out as *ad hoc* bedside teaching. Short educational sessions on different topics like pain management were arranged and written support material developed and distributed. The inevitable resistance following the introduction of change into a system, like a NICU, was sought overcome by anchoring the intervention in the existing organization, and securing the support of leaders and senior clinicians. Additionally half-day seminars on implementing change, personal and organizational reactions to change, and the change process were provided. All nurses, but few of the physicians attended the change seminars.

The project groups met regularly during the intervention period and supported each other through the discussion of progress and problems. In the second half of the intervention period, a new procedure for blood collection replaced heel-stick with venous blood sampling. Prior to implementation, all staff received education regarding venous blood sampling. After sufficient demonstration, a group of 4-6 nurses started practicing. When they had acquired sufficient practical skills, they tutored a new group of nurses. By the end of the intervention period, almost all members of the nursing staff mastered the new procedure.

3. Evaluation

The pre-test questionnaires were distributed at the start of the one-day neonatal pain-management seminars prior to the intervention in spring 2003. After receiving information about the study, attendants each received a copy of the questionnaire and were given 20 minutes to complete it. Respondents were seated in a classroom style, to give everyone sufficient privacy. No one refused to participate or returned a blank questionnaire. All participants were asked to mark their name on a staff list to indicate their participation; the questionnaires did not include any information that could later identify the respondent. The participants were asked not to discuss the content of the questionnaire or the seminars with colleagues. Staff not present were approached after the seminars and asked to complete the questionnaire. If the questionnaire was not returned, one reminder was given. The answers were analyzed and the results disseminated back to the staff during the first part of the intervention period. At the end of the intervention period, 2 years later, the same questionnaire were distributed among the staff for a new evaluation of practice. Each member of staff received a questionnaire and an enclosed letter asking them to complete the questionnaire. Completed questionnaires were sent or delivered to the project manager and respondents were asked to mark their name on a staff list placed in the staff office in the NICU. One reminder was given to non-responders after approx. 2 weeks.

Statistical Analyses

Data on background variables at the two time points were compared using the χ^2 test, except for age (t test). The results for the two time points were compared for each question (e.g. procedure painfulness, current use of pharmacological agents etc.) and procedure (e.g. endotracheal intubation, insertion of chest tube, insertion of gavage tube etc.) using the Mann–Whitney U test. When a significant difference was detected, respondents were divided into subgroups (nurses and physicians) and a *post hoc* test was performed. P ≤ 0.05 was considered statistically significant.

RESULTS

Procedure Painfulness

A significant change (2003 vs. 2005) in the respondents' perception of procedure painfulness was observed for 4/10 procedures (Figure 1).

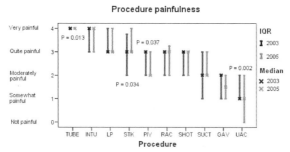

Figure 1.

The nurses changed their views as follows: in 2005 the insertion of a chest tube ($P = 0.006$) and the heel stick ($P = 0.039$) were considered more painful, and the insertion of a peripheral intravenous line ($P = 0.015$) and the insertion of an umbilical catheter ($P = 0.001$) were perceived less painful. There were no significant changes in physicians' perceptions between the two measurement events.

Actual Use of Pharmacological Agents

Although the respondents reported an infrequent use of pharmacological agents for most procedures on both measurement occasions, a significant increase was reported for 5/10 procedures (Figure 2). The changes in the nurses answers were significant for the procedures insertion of a chest tube ($P = 0,005$) and insertion of a peripheral intravenous line ($P = 0.013$), while significant changes among the physicians were found for the procedures lumbar puncture ($P = 0,004$) and insertion of a radial or tibial arterial catheter ($P = 0,008$). There were no significant changes on the subgroup level for the procedure tracheal suctioning.

Optimal Use of Pharmacological Agents

The respondents' answers on the post-test indicated that they would use pharmacological agents most frequently for those procedures with the highest ratings for pain, except the heel stick (Figure 3). Physicians' perceptions did not change between the two time points, but there were a significant decrease in the nurses' answers regarding the use of pharmacological agents for the procedures heel stick ($P = 0.001$), insertion of a gavage tube ($P = 0.002$), and insertion of an umbilical catheter ($P = 0.001$).

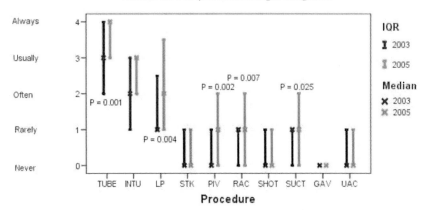

Medians and interquartile ranges (IQR) of physicians' and nurses' answers in 2003 (N=73) and 2005 (N=67).

Figure 2.

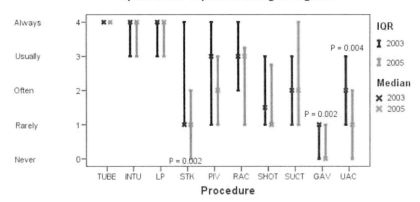

Medians and interquartile ranges (IQR) of physicians' and nurses' answers in 2003 (N=73) and 2005 (N=67).

Figure 3.

Actual Use of Comfort Measures

The respondents' rating of the actual use of comfort measures on the post-test exceeded "often" (median ≥ 2) for all procedures except intubation (Figure 4). Whereas the nurses answers indicated an increased use of comfort measures during the heel stick ($P = 0.034$) and the insertion of a gavage tube ($P = 0.001$), there were no significant changes over time in physicians' answers.

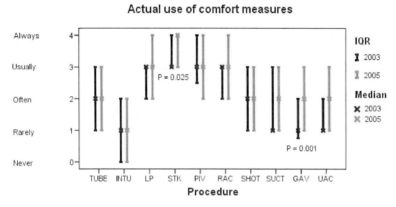

TUBE=insertion of chest tube, INTU=endotracheal intubation, LP=lumbar puncture, STK=heel stick, PIV=insertion of peripheral intravenous line, RAC=insertion of radial or tibial arterial catheter, SHOT=intramuscular injection, SUCT=tracheal suctioning, GAV=insertion of gavage tube and UAC=insertion of umbilical catheter.

Medians and interquartile ranges (IQR) of physicians' and nurses' answers in 2003 (N=73) and 2005 (N=67).

Figure 4.

Optimal Use of Comfort Measures

At both measurement occasions, physicians and nurses indicated that comfort measures should be used more frequently than what was actually done in current practice. No significant changes in reporting of performance of single procedures were detected (Figure 5).

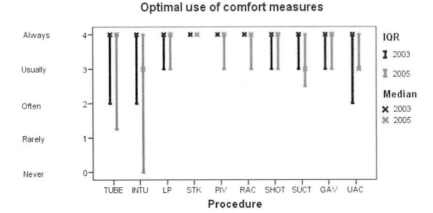

TUBE=insertion of chest tube, INTU=endotracheal intubation, LP=lumbar puncture, STK=heel stick, PIV=insertion of peripheral intravenous line, RAC=insertion of radial or tibial arterial catheter, SHOT=intramuscular injection, SUCT=tracheal suctioning, GAV=insertion of gavage tube and UAC=insertion of umbilical catheter.

Medians and interquartile ranges (IQR) of physicians' and nurses' answers in 2003 (N=73) and 2005 (N=67).

Figure 5.

DISCUSSION

This paper reports on the differences of clinicians' perceptions concerning the treatment of procedural pain in neonates, before and after the implementation of new pain management strategies in two NICUs in southern Norway. Clinicians' answers indicated a slight increase in the use of pharmacological agents after the intervention. Only the nurses reported changes in their views of procedure painfulness, the actual use of comfort measures, and the perceived optimal treatment for procedural pain. The intervention did not generate enhanced accordance in the perceptions of physicians and nurses.

This study has several weaknesses. Most important is the lack of control groups. The observed changes may have been influenced by factors other than the intervention. For example, during the intervention period, nurses from both units participated in a 60 h external competence program for neonatal nurses, which included a 3 h session on neonatal pain and pain management. However, its content was mainly in line with the first education program provided as part of the intervention. Furthermore, in 2004, the Norwegian Pediatric Pain Society was founded during a meeting initiated by the pediatric department at one of the study sites. In general, there was growing attention to pediatric pain issues among Norwegian health personnel during this period. Another limitation is the sample sizes. They were small; especially the numbers of physicians, and thus, the statistical power is low. The strength of the study is the small turnover in the clinical staff at both hospitals during the project period, where 2/3 of the respondents to the pre-test questionnaire in 2003 also responded to the post-test questionnaire in 2005.

The elements of the intervention were based on the theoretical underpinnings described in the introduction. Looking back, this framework has been important for two reasons: First, it explains why there is no direct link between knowledge and practice, and second, it helped in choosing the different elements included in the study, resulting in a multifaceted intervention with a strong emphasis on both knowledge transfer and actions related to the social setting.

The respondents' views on procedure painfulness and the optimal treatment of procedural pain are largely consistent with international guidelines [21] and previous studies [15]. The respondents' different professional backgrounds may also influence their answers. The pharmacological treatment of pain is the physicians' responsibility, although treatment is mainly administered by nurses. The nurses' answers on the actual use of pharmacological agents can be viewed as an assessment of the physicians' practice and not their own, whereas the physicians' answers reflect an evaluation of their own practice. For the assessment of actual use of comfort measures, it probably worked the other way around. The differences in the nurses and physicians' answers may reflect the extent to which they consider themselves responsible for the treatment in question, rather than accurately reflecting actual pain-management practice in the two units studied. Unfortunately, self assessment of practice appears to be a weak proxy measure of actual practice [21].

The respondents' views on procedure painfulness and the optimal treatment of procedural pain were largely consistent with international guidelines [21] and previous studies [7, 15]. Respondents' perceptions showed only minor changes over two years, indicating that these beliefs are relatively stable. However, the changes observed are noteworthy. Only the nurses rated heel stick as more painful after the intervention period and only the nurses were involved in changing the procedure of blood sampling. The nurses' answers in the post-test were probably influenced by multiple factors; their involvement in the change of practice, an increased knowledge of the pain associated with blood sampling and their own observations during the change in the procedure. Prior to the intervention, the nurses performed the heel stick or assisted phlebotomists in performing the procedure. Based on the new method, the nurses were trained to perform venous punctures for blood sampling and had the opportunity to observe first-hand the differences in the neonates' behavioral responses towards heel-stick and venous puncture. The procedure detailed the environmental and behavioral interventions that should be applied during blood sampling, and the nurses' answers indicated a significant increase in the use of comfort measures during heel-stick sampling. Knowledge about the available pharmacological treatments for the different procedures was disseminated throughout the intervention period. No appropriate pharmacological treatment is available for the heel-stick procedure. This knowledge was reflected in the nurses' answers, which indicated a significant drop in the optimal use of pharmacological agents for this procedure. It indicates a connection between personal involvements in the change process and changes in beliefs and practice.

The differences between the nurses and physicians' perceptions persisted over the study period. The nurses still perceived the various procedures to be more painful than did the physicians, and nurses would still use both comfort measures and pharmacological agents more frequently compared with the physicians. Different education, different roles, and different areas of responsibility are plausible explanations. The answers of both groups indicated an increase in the pharmacological treatment of neonatal pain, but only the nurses reported changes in the use of comfort measures. Both methods were included in the education program and in the guidelines, but it is likely that more emphasis was put on the use of pharmacological agents. Another possible explanation is that whereas pharmacological treatments are concrete, clearly defined, measurable, and documented in the infants' medical charts, comfort measures are less clearly defined, adaptable both in regard to the professional carrying out the procedure and to the patient receiving care, and not documented in a systematic manner. The differences in the physicians and nurses' views on the use of comfort measures may reflect the extent to which comfort is provided. The nurses' answers indicated a significant increase in the use of comfort measures only for procedures that were carried out independently by the nurses. It seems that authority is an important factor for the implementation of evidence-based practice. Physicians are the main decision makers in the hospital. It might be so that the nurses adapt their practice to fit in with the physicians' perception in situations where both professions work together. Even when the use of comfort measures is considered the nurses' responsibility, it seems that the nurses will not change their practice if the physicians do not actively support this change.

It appears that the intervention, although designed for a multiprofessional group, influenced the nurses more than the physicians. This may be the result of basic differences between the two professions and/or the specific characteristics of the intervention. In a recent study of factors influencing practice change in the emergency department, physician leadership was identified as a driving force in the change process. Physicians were viewed as the main decision makers and their approval as a necessary success criterion [23]. The intervention reported in the current study was initiated and led by a nurse. Although physician cooperation was sought in all phases of the intervention, the origin in nursing rather than in medicine may have influenced how both nurses and physicians chose to get involved in the change process. Another study showed that physicians and nurses view the use of guidelines differently. While nurses advocated the use of guidelines, physicians were more likely to reject them and rely on their clinical judgment and the unwritten rules of their profession [24]. This is a potential explanation to why the current intervention, which was heavily based on the implementation of new guidelines, appears to have targeted the nurses better than the physicians. Future research should investigate if and how the specific characteristics of an intervention influence nurses and physicians differently, and explore whether it is beneficial to plan interventions differently according to the profession of the recipients.

Despite the performance of a multifaceted intervention to support evidence-based practice, the overall results point clearly to the difficulties in applying evidence to practice. Apart from a slight increase in the actual use of pharmacological agents, the intervention did not result in any main changes in the treatment of procedural pain in neonates. The context, including how the different professions perceive and respond to a knowledge translation intervention and how they collaborate, appears to be a major challenge in the implementation of evidence into practice. Change is not an easy or straightforward process. It is necessary to gain a better understanding of the main factors that influence the change process. Clinical research is of little value if the results cannot be translated into clinical practice to benefit patients and practitioners.

ACKNOWLEDGMENT

The authors would like to thank Fran Lang Porter for the permission to use questions from her survey and Martin Svendsen for statistical advice.

This article is based on results from a project that were financed with the aid of EXTRA funds from the Norwegian Foundation for Health and Rehabilitation.

REFERENCES

[1]   Stevens BJ, Anand KJS, McGrath PJ. An overview of pain in neonates and infants. In: Anand KJS, Stevens BJ, McGrath PJ, editors. *Pain in neonates and infants.* 3rd edition. Philadelphia: Elsevier; 2007: 1-7.

[2]   Andersen RD, Greve-Isdahl M, Jylli L. The opinions of clinical staff regarding neonatal procedural pain in two Norwegian neonatal intensive care units. *Acta Paediatr.* 2007;96(7):1000-1003.

[3]   Wallin L. Knowledge Utilization in Swedish Neonatal Nursing. Studies on Guideline Implementation, Change Processes and Contextual Factors. *Doctoral thesis.* Uppsala: Uppsala University; 2003.

[4]   Fitzgerald M. Development of the peripheral and spinal pain system. In: Anand KJS, Stevens BJ, McGrath PJ, editors. *Pain in Neonates.* 2nd Revised and Enlarged Edition. Amsterdam: Elsevier; 2000. p. 9-22.

[5]   Anand KJ, Hickey PR. Pain and its effects in the human neonate and fetus. *N. Engl. J. Med.* 1987;317(21):1321-9.

[6]   McGrath PJ, Unruh AM. The social context of neonatal pain. *Clin. Perinatol.* 2002;29(3):555-72.

[7]   Simons SH, van Dijk M, Anand KS, Roofthooft D, van Lingen RA, Tibboel D. Do we still hurt newborn babies? A prospective study of procedural pain and analgesia in neonates. *Arch. Pediatr. Adolesc. Med.* 2003;157(11):1058-64.

[8]   Stevens BJ, Riddell RRP, Oberlander TE, Gibbins S. Assessment of pain in neonates and infants. In: Anand KJS, Stevens BJ, McGrath PJ, editors. *Pain in neonates and infants.* 3rd edition. Philadelphia: Elsevier; 2007: 67-90.

[9]   Lago P, Guadagni A, Merazzi D, Ancora G, Bellieni CV, Cavazza A. Pain management in the neonatal intensive care unit: a national survey in Italy. *Paediatr. Anaesth.* 2005;15(11):925-31.

[10] Harrison D, Loughnan P, Johnston L. Pain assessment and procedural pain management practices in neonatal units in Australia. *J. Paediatr. Child Health* 2006;42(1-2):6-9.

[11] Rohrmeister K, Kretzer V, Berger A, Haiden N, Kohlhauser C, Pollak A. Pain and stress management in the Neonatal Intensive Care Unit--a national survey in Austria. *Wien Klin. Wochenschr* 2003;115(19-20):715-9.

[12] Anand KJ, Craig KD. New perspectives on the definition of pain. *Pain* 1996;67(1):3-6; discussion 209-11.

[13] Franck LS, Lawhon G. Environmental and behavioral strategies to prevent and manage neonatal pain. In: Anand KJS, Stevens BJ, McGrath PJ, editors. *Pain in Neonates.* 2nd Revised and Enlarged Edition. Amsterdam: Elsevier; 2000. p. 203-216.

[14] Shah V, Ohlsson A. Venepuncture versus heel lance for blood sampling in term neonates. *Cochrane Database Syst Rev.* 2007(4):CD001452.

[15] Porter FL, Wolf CM, Gold J, Lotsoff D, Miller JP. Pain and pain management in newborn infants: a survey of physicians and nurses. *Pediatrics* 1997;100(4):626-32.

[16] Grunau RE. Long-term consequences of pain in human neonates. In: Anand KJ, Stevens B, McGrath PJ, editors. *Pain in Neonates*, 2nd Revised and Enlarged Edition. Amsterdam: Elsevier; 2000. p. 55-76.

[17] Eccles M, Mittman B. Welcome to Implementation Science. In: *Implementation Science.* 2006;1(1):1.

[18] Grimshaw JM, Thomas RE, MacLennan G, Fraser C, Ramsay CR, Vale L, et al. Effectiveness and efficiency of guideline dissemination and implementation strategies. *Health Technol Assess* 2004;8(6):iii-iv, 1-72.

[19] Estabrooks CA, Floyd JA, Scott-Findlay S, O'Leary KA, Gushta M. Individual determinants of research utilization: a systematic review. *J. Adv. Nurs.* 2003;43(5):506-20.

[20] Atkinson RL, Atkinson RC, Smith EE, Bem DJ. Introduction to Psychology. Eleventh edition. Forth Worth: Harcourt Brace Jovanovitch College Publishers; 1993.

[21] Anand KJ. Consensus statement for the prevention and management of pain in the newborn. *Arch. Pediatr. Adolesc.* Med. 2001;155(2):173-80.

[22] Larsson BA, Gradin M, Lind V, Selander B. [Swedish guidelines for prevention and treatment of pain in newborn infants]. In Swedish. *Lakartidningen* 2002;99(17):1946-9.

[23] Hurley KF, Sargeant J, Duffy J, Sketris I, Sinclair D, Ducharme J. Perceptual reasons for resistance to change in the emergency department

use of holding chambers for children with asthma. *Ann. Emerg. Med.* 2008;51(1):70-7.

[24] McDonald R, Waring J, Harrison S, Walshe K, Boaden R. Rules and guidelines in clinical practice: a qualitative study in operating theatres of doctors' and nurses' views. *Qual. Saf Health Care* 2005;14(4):290-4

In: Pregnancy and Infants
Editor: Tsisana Shartava

ISBN 978-1-61209-132-7
© 2011 Nova Science Publishers, Inc.

Chapter 6

BREASTFEEDING DURING CRISES AND EMERGENCIES

Iftikhar Alam[1], Parvez Iqbal Paracha[1] and Safia Begum[2]*

1. Department of Human Nutrition, Faculty of Nutrition Sciences
Agriculture University Peshawar NWFP Pakistan
2. Dertment of Human Development Studies, College of Home Econoics
Peshawar University, Peshawar NWFP Pakistan

ABSTRACT

Data for the present work were based on electronic search of research studies published on the subject. The literature suggests that chances of malnutrition in infants considerably increase during natural disasters and crisis situations. In such emergencies, helping mothers successfully initiate and continue breastfeeding becomes even more crucial.

Children in vulnerable situations have special needs for infection-fighting factors, optimal nutrition, reliable food source and comfort; all

* DAAD Scholar for PhD, Tübingen Aging and Tumor Immunology group, Sektion fürTransplantationsimmunologie und Immunohämatologie, University of Tübingen, Zentrum für Medizinische Forschung, Waldhörnlestraße 22, 72072Tübingen, Germany, ialamk@yahoo.com

these can be ensured only by breastfeeding. Usually the water sources are contaminated during emergencies and if used for dilution of powdered milk and/or washing of nipples and bottles, this water can cause irreversible health damage to the infants.

In contrast, human milk provides ample hydration and spares infants exposure to contaminated water due to destruction in emergencies. As rate of infections increases during emergencies; infants who are not breastfed will be more susceptible to infections and other illnesses. Consequently, they will be more likely to require hospitalization and to die in the first year of life, in fact, considerably costing the families and community. Mothers warrant extra support during crises; which demands for rapidly keeping their infants with them and providing space where they can feel comfortable nursing. Mothers delivering during the crisis should be encouraged and helped to initiate breastfeeding immediately after birth and to exclusive breastfeed for approximately 6 months.

Those mothers who recently stopped breastfeeding due to stress should be assisted to relactate. Misconceptions and fears leading to stop and/or minimize breastfeeding must be dispelled with accurate information. Wherever and whenever needed suitable arrangements for wet nursing must be made ensuring optimal infant nutritional requirements. Beside, proper feeding the mother is the safest, most effective way to ensure adequate infant nutrition during emergencies.

INTRODUCTION

Breastfeeding in emergency situations and other natural disasters becomes even more important. It is because the existing health risks of bottle and formula feeding in emergencies are greatly increased due to poor hygiene, possible contaminated water supply, lack of proper storage, limited fuel for formula heating and crowding etc. Breastfeeding is crucial for the survival of the children in emergency situations as it provides protection against inadequacy and contamination of complementary foods and a number of diseases an infections (Rautava and Walker, 2009; Mead, 2008; DeWald and Fountain, 2006) and reduces the risks of sudden infant death syndrome (Vennemann, *et al.,* 2009). It also provides an opportunity of the bonding, warmth and care by the mother to the baby, much needed in such circumstances.

Emergency situations are usually initially confusing and chaotic. To determine who needs what is an essential early step. For protecting and supporting breastfeeding, the first step is to identify infants who are or should be breastfed and further noting any infants who are temporarily or permanently without their mother (Moss *et al.,* 2006; UNICEF/UNHCR 1994; Sapir 1993; Ressler 1988; Williamson 1988). In global emergency and relief situations, it is important to breastfeed infants and young children as artificial feeding in these conditions is difficult and hazardous and leads to increased infant mortality rates (WHO/UNICEF, 2002; IBFAN, 2001). Conversely, human milk is the natural nutrition for all infants (American Academy of Pediatrics, 2004). Evidence suggests that breastfeeding decreases risks for many diseases in infants (Ip *et al.,* 2007; Horta *et al.,* 2007).

Some misconceptions about breastfeeding in emergencies often lead to high levels of infant mortality. A number of cultural, religious, economical and other factors may affect the practice of breastfeeding (Thulier, 2009). It is assumed that mothers who are malnourished and under stress during emergencies can not and should not breastfeed their infants. However, it has been proved that even women who are malnourished and under stress can produce plenty of quality milk for their babies (Kawasaki, 2005). Some of the obstacles to initiation and continuation of breastfeeding include insufficient prenatal education about breastfeeding, disruptive maternity care practices, and lack of family and broad societal support (AAP, 2002). Some complex emergencies are associated with large numbers of unaccompanied children (Sapir, 1993), and these children have special needs which should be addressed with utmost priority (UNICEF/UNHCR 1994; Ressler 1988; Williamson 1988).

A vast scientific literature demonstrates the substantial health, social and economic importance of breastfeeding, including lower infant and young child morbidity and mortality from diarrhea and other infectious diseases (Cattaneo *et al.,*2006; Chen and Rogan, 2004; Jones *et al.,* 2003; Cunningham *et al.,*1991). The health and nutritional advantages can be maximized by 1) exclusively breastfeeding in the first 6 months (Kramer and Kakuma, 2004) and, 2) extending the duration of breastfeeding into the second year and beyond (Mortensen *et al.,*2002). It has been recommended that exclusive breastfeeding of infants for the first 6 months, after which mothers are recommended to continue breastfeeding; in combination with suitably nutritious and safe complementary foods – semi-solid and solid foods –until their children are 2 years of age or older (WHO/UNICEF, 2002).

Addressing the health needs of children in complex emergencies is critical to the success of relief efforts and requires effective and coordinated interventions. To make breastfeeding a success during emergency situations, compliance with internationally recognized best practice guidelines and directives is essential (WHO, 2003; WHO/UNICEF, 1997; and strict measures have to be taken to ensure breastfeeding during such situation (EU Project 2004; Cattaneo and Bussetti, 2001; Hogan, 2001; Bradley, 1992; Popkin *et al.*,1991; Rea, 1990; Rea and Berquo, 1990). The goals of Healthy People 2010 for breastfeeding are an initiation rate of 75% and continuation rate of 50% at 6 months and 25% at 12 months after delivery (U.S. Department of Health and Human Services, 2000) and emergency situations are no exception.

ANALYSIS OF THE SITUATION

Humanity has witnessed a number of devastating emergency situations in forms of natural disasters, famine and wars in the recent past. The emergency situations have always been a challenge to humanity, regarding the health and feeding of the children of breastfeeding age, in particular. The destruction caused by theses in terms of health loss is sometime irreversible.

Diseases and Infections

Diarrheal diseases, acute respiratory infections, measles, malaria, and severe malnutrition in children are very common in emergency situations (Shears *et al.*, 1985; Porter *et al.*,1990; Toole and Waldman 1997; Siddique *et al.*,1995; Salama et al 2001; Rowland *et al.*, 2001; Peterson *et al.*, 2001; Roberts *et al.*, 2001; Swerdlo *et al.*, 2002; Black *et al.*, 2003; Bloland and Williams 2003) Examples of other infectious diseases include outbreaks of poliomyelitis (Valente *et al.*, 2000), cutaneous leishmaniasis (Rowland *et al.*,1997), meningococcal meningitis (Santaniello and Hunter 2000) etc.Tuberculosis can spread rapidly during emergency situations due to overcrowding and poor nutritional and dietary practices (Bar and Menzies 1994).

Mortality and Morbidity

High proportions of mortality and morbidity in emergencies are in children. A review of child mortality in various refugee camps in the early 1980's reported a mortality rate more than twice as high in children younger than 5 years of age (32.6 per 10,000 per day) than the overall crude mortality rate (Toole and Waldman 1990). In a refugee camp in Bangladesh, most deaths occurred among infants (640 per 1000 per year) and children (357 per 1000 per year) (Khan and Munshi 1983). The overall mortality among Ethiopian refugees in Sudan in February 1985 was 8.9 per 10,000 persons per day, but was 22 per 10,000 per day for children less than 5 years of age (Shears 1991). Among refugees in Honduras between 1984 and 1987, deaths in infants accounted for 42% of all deaths, and deaths in children younger than 5 years for 54% of all deaths (Desenclos et al., 1990). A survey conducted during the 1991 Kurdish refugee crisis found that two thirds of all deaths occurred in children less than 5 years, and half were among infants younger than 1 year (Yip et al., 1993). The Gulf war and trade sanctions were estimated to have caused a threefold increase in mortality among Iraqi children younger than 5 years of age, resulting in an excess mortality of 46,900 children between January and August 1991 (Ascherio et al., 1992). Recently in the Congo crisis, one-third of the total number of deaths consisted of children less than five years of age. It was estimated that 75% of children born during the war, died or would die before their second birthday (O'Conor et al., 2001).

Unaccompanied Children

Emergency situations often leave a large number of unaccompanied children with special health-care needs (UNCF/UNHCR 1994; Ressler et al.,1988). These are usually older children, however, may be abandoned infants (Spair 1993). Extremely high mortality rates were documented among unaccompanied Rwandan refugee children after arrival in Goma, Democratic Republic of the Congo (Dowell 1995). Most deaths (85%) occurred more than 2 days after arrival at relief centers, suggesting that early and appropriate care could have significantly reduced mortality. The war in the Congo resulted in large numbers of unaccompanied children, some of whom were not yet weaned from the breast. Unaccompanied children have suffered the highest mortality rates of all vulnerable groups, ranging between 20 and 120 deaths per 10,000 persons per day. In Rwanda, it was estimated that 1,800 unaccompanied children were present out of 450,000 Hutu refugees. Of these, about 50 were below the age of 2 years (Puoane et al., 2001). In Eastern Zaire, young babies were found alive and abandoned at massacre sites. Other mothers were sick or malnourished and died during the trip.

Malnutrition in Emergencies

Malnutrition and micronutrient deficiencies are very common in emergencies and these contribute substantially to child morbidity and mortality (Toole and Waldman 1997; CDC 1992). The median prevalence of acute malnutrition among children less than 5 years of age in internally displaced and conflict-affected populations between 1988 and 1995 was 31% and was as high as 80% in the Sudan in 1993 (Toole and Waldman, 1997). More recent surveys have found similar high prevalence rates of acute malnutrition in children in complex emergencies. A nutritional assessment survey of children in the North Korea in 1997, found a prevalence of acute malnutrition as high as 33% in some regions of the country (Katona-Apte Mokdd, 1998). Wasting was estimated to have contributed to 72% of all deaths among children younger than 5 years of age during a famine in Ethiopia in 2000 (Salama *et al.,* 2001). Deficiencies of iron and vitamin A are more common and severe in refugee or displaced children (Weise and de Benoist 2002). In addition, uncommon micronutrient deficiencies, such as scurvy (vitamin C deficiency), pellagra (niacin and/or tryptophan), and beriberi (thiamine), may affect large populations in complex emergencies. A strong association between severe wasting in children and high mortality rates in refugee populations has been reported (Mason 2002). Besides severe malnutrition, mild to moderate malnutrition is likely to be a significant underlying cause of death in children in emergencies (Rice *et al.,* 2000; Pelletier *et al.,* 1995).

NUTRITIONAL REQUIREMENTS OF CHILDREN AND BREASTFEEDING

The importance of breastfeeding in the diet of infants and toddlers varies with the age of the child. Younger children caused the greatest difficulties with regard to feeding, as they required exclusive breastfeeding if they were to have a chance of survival (Puoane *et al.,* 2001). For infants 6–12 months of age, weaning foods should be added to the diet in a gradually increasing manner. Breast milk provides the major part of energy requirements of the infant (Stephen and George, 2009). Research shows that breast milk supplies 85% of an infant's caloric intake at six months of age, 63% at nine months of age and 38% at 12 months of age (Dewy *et al.* 2001). However, a study in Honduras showed that at one year of age, approximately 80% of the infant's caloric intake still came from breast milk (Cohen *et al.,* 1995).

Advocacy for Breastfeeding during Emergencies and Crisis

Breastfeeding in emergencies and conflicts can best be advocated through its cost effectiveness and its biological significance. All policies, planning and strategies developed should adhere to these two points in order to minimize infants' mortality and morbidity as a result of malnutrition during emergencies.

Breastfeeding is a cost effective approach as it eliminates health service costs for free supplies of infant formula (Food Safety Authority of Ireland (FSAI), 2005). It has been reported that a higher rate and duration of breastfeeding is associated with reduced cost for the family, the health care system and society in general (Baby Milk Action, 2000; Ball and Wright, 1999; US Dept of Commerce, 1999; Montgomery and Splett, 1997; Tuttle and Dewey, 1996; Baumslag and Michels, 1995). Breastfeeding reduces the health care costs for care attributable to childhood illnesses (Radford, 2002; Weimer, 2001; Ball and Wright, 1999; Drane, 1997; Riordan, 1997). Moreover, it also reduces hospital maternity costs for teats and formula purchases (Department of Health and Children (DOHC), 2003). In addition, breastfeeding reduces environmental costs as a result of the reduction in packaging, transport costs and wasteful by-products of both the production and use of artificial feeding (Webster, 2000).

The family planning might be of great help to maintain maternal health during emergencies. Mothers who breastfeed show earlier return to pre-pregnancy weight   (Dewey *et al.,* 1993), increased self-confidence and enhanced bonding with their infants (Kuzela *et al.,* 1990). Delayed resumption of fertility for most women, thereby assisting in family planning is also closely associate with breastfeeding (McNeilly, 1993).

The relief workers working in emergencies should know the importance of breast milk. Only then they can advocate breastfeeding effectively by translating the scientific language into the layman language regarding the benefits of breastfeeding. The relief workers should now and must be able to convey following benefits to the target community in gneral and t the nursing mothers in particular.

- Breastfeeding reduces risks of infections (Rautava and Walker, 2009; Mead, 2008) and risks of sudden infant death syndrome (Vennemann, *et al.,* 2009).
- Breastfeeding reduces the severity and incidence of diarrhea (Chung *et al.,* 2008), which is one of the major causes of mortality among infants and young children in developing countries.
- Breastfeeding reduces the risk of lower respiratory infections (Bachrach et 2003), urinary tract infection (Marild *et al.,* 2004), invasive bacterial infection (Goldman, 1993), ear infections (Duncan *et al.,*1993), otitis media (Scariati *et al.,* 2008) and pneumonia/asthma (Kull *et al.,* 2004).
- Breastfeeding may protect metabolic diseases (Pettitt *et al.,*1997), necrotizing enterocolitis (Gorman *et al.,* 1996), Type 1 and Type 2 diabetes, (Owen *et al.,* 2006), obesity (Arenz *et al.,* 2004) and inflammatory bowel disease (Klement *et al.,* 2004).
- Breastfeeding may protect infants from childhood leukemia (Kwan *et al.,* 2004), chronic digestive and respiratory diseases (Oddy *et al.,*1999; Cunningham, 1995), Crohn's disease (Klement *et al.,* 2004; Cunningham, 1995), celiac disease (Greco *et al.,* 1997), childhood cancer (Shu *et al.,*1999), allergic disease (Oddy *et al.,* 1999) and cardiovascular disease (Owen *et al.,* 2002).
- Breastfed infants show a better response to vaccines (Pabst, 1989).
- Breastfeeding can decrease bleeding and help maintain the firmness of the uterus of a new mother (American College of Nurse-Midwives [ACNM], 2003).
- The benefits of the infection-fighting properties of colostrum hold an increased value during times of disaster (ACNM, 2003).

Misconceptions and Myths about Breastfeeding

The practice of breastfeeding is greatly affected by certain myths (Hyman and Stanner, 2004). People affected by wars or natural disasters often have to live in crowded and insanitary conditions. Their access to food and health care services may also be restricted. In these settings. the danger of diarrhea and other infections is great. This means that during emergencies breastfeeding becomes even more important in protecting infant health. Experience of relief operations in a range of countries has shown that anxieties about breastfeeding were most common in countries where artificial feeding was widespread before the emergency began. Even during war and famine in Ethiopia and Sudan, inability to breastfeed was much less commonly reported than in recent emergencies in Iraq, Eastern Europe and the former Soviet Union. This difference suggests that cultural factors are more important in influencing breastfeeding than the emergency itself. As countries become more industrialized, artificial infant feeding is often introduced and breastfeeding skills tend to be lost. In many cases, inaccurate and out-of-date information about breastfeeding replaces traditional knowledge.

Cultures around the world have their own myths surrounding breastfeeding. These myths are often damaging because they do not permit for mother and child to have a successful breastfeeding experience. It is not known where all these myths come from but it is important to address them promptly so that a successful breastfeeding practice may take place during emergency situations. The health team workers working in emergency situations must be aware of them. They should also have ample scientific answers to these misconceptions. Only then an effective relief strategy can be developed and implemented to promote breastfeeding in emergencies.

Myth 1: Women under stress in emergency situations cannot breastfeed. There is not enough milk due to stress and anxiety, so bottle-feeding would be a better solution for both the child and the mother.

Truth: Poor milk supply is closely related with infrequent feeding and/or poor latch-on and positioning. Both of these are usually due to inadequate information provided to the breastfeeding mother. Suckling problem on the part of the infant may also negatively affect milk supply. Stress and anxiety are rarely the causes of milk supply problems (Hill 2005; Heinig 2005; Dusdieker 1990, Woolridge 1995).

Myth 2: Malnourished women don't produce enough milk OR the mother has recently lost weight and she has not been eating well for the last few days can not produce enough milk.

Truth: Milk volume is the result of infant demand rather than a reflection of maternal capacity (Kawasaki, 2005; Daly and Hartmann 1995). A woman's diet will not usually limit her ability to produce sufficient breast milk. It is, however, recommended that proper nutritional care of a lactating woman should be taken of to ensure proper milk supply and optimal health status of the mother.

Myth 3: In emergencies as the mother can no longer afford to buy fresh fruits and vegetables. Her diet consists mainly of food aid rations. Surely if she eats a diet of such poor quality she will produce milk of poor quality. And/or the mother is anemic; feeding her baby might cause the baby to become anemic too.

Truth: Regarding mother's nutrition, women have produced very adequate milk supplies on very inadequate diets. Research has shown that mothers even with mild malnutrition status can produce an adequate supply of good quality milk. Even in famine conditions, milk production is slightly effected (Perez-Escamilla 1995; Prentice 1994; Kelly 1993).

Myth 4: Once Breastfeeding Has Stopped, It cannot be resumed.

Truth: For some mothers and babies, once breastfeeding has stopped, it may be resumed successfully. With an adequate relactation technique and support, it is possible to help mothers and their babies to restart breastfeeding after their babies have been switched to infant formula. This is sometimes vital in an emergency (Kawasaki, 2005; American Academy of Pediatrics, 2004).

Myth 5: A baby with diarrhea should not be breastfed.

Truth: Breastfeeding is rather very good during diarrhea (Chung *et al.,* 2008; Dewey *et al.,*1995). Real causes of diarrhea should be corrected. Stopping breastfeeding during when the infant is suffering from diarrhea may worsen his/her illness further.

Difficulties of Mothers during Emergencies: Mothers are greatly affected by emergencies and crisis situations. The relief workers should appreciate their problems. At the same time they should provide the necessary support for the solutions of these problems. Some of the difficulties faced by mothers reported in the literature are lack of privacy, not having proper shelter, fear of future emergency, grief of loss, dejection, sleeplessness, no motivation, a feeling that they are not of the priority (Breastfeeding Promotion Network of India (BPNI), 2005), etc.

Maternal Nutritional Care

An increase in food intake can be a source of energy and protein to meet the increased energy requirement during breastfeeding. Breastfeeding women are generally reported to increase their energy intake to, at least partly, accommodate their increased energy expenditure (Todd and Parnell 1994). However, evidence from developing countries suggests that some women do not increase their energy intake but still produce adequate milk (Prentice et al 1980).

Other aspects to consider in the energy balance of breastfeeding women are changes in BMR and diet-induced thermogenesis. There is some evidence that energy savings occur through these mechanisms, although a recent review of the research suggests that they are not thought to be significant in well-nourished women (Institute of Medicine 2002).

In general a diet containing fresh fruits and vegetables, dry nuts, whole cereals and iron fortified cereal products, dairy products as source of calcium and vitamin A are recommended.

Optimal Breastfeeding Practices in Emergencies

The first step in relief efforts is to create policies that make breastfeeding information a priority. New way to help implement theses policies is to find women in the affected areas who have breastfeeding knowledge and the skills to help others breastfeed and enlist their assistance (Kelly 1993 manual).

Community-based breastfeeding facilities can teach appropriate latch-on skills, counsel mothers on overcoming common breastfeeding problems. In the following are summarized some points given in published researches, which should be observed strictly for optimal breastfeeding practices during emergencies (United States Breastfeeding Committee, 2008; Ip et al 2007; LLL 2006; manual Infant Feeding in Emergency, 2005; WHO 2004; Pediatric Nutrition Handbook 2004; WHO 2001; WHO 2000).

1. Help mothers initiate breastfeeding within an hour of birth.
2. Ensure effective infant positioning (latch-on)
3. Show mothers how to breastfeed, and how to maintain lactation even if they should be separated from their infants.
4. Ensure exclusive breastfeeding for 6 months of age and sustained breastfeeding well into the second year of life or beyond
5. Increased breastfeeding frequency and continued feeding during illness and after illness for catch up growth.
6. Encourage relactation
7. If needed, use hand expressed milk for feeding
8. Continuation of breastfeeding after beginning the addition of appropriate weaning foods at 6 months of age
9. If needed, make arrangements for wet nursing to breastfeeding infants.

The Relief Agencies Should Make Sure the Following

1. The quantity, distribution and use of breast-milk substitutes and artificial teats (also called dummies or soothers) at emergencies should be strictly controlled.
2. A nutritionally adequate breast-milk substitute should be available and fed by cup only to those infants who have to be fed on breast-milk substitutes.
3. Because the number of caregivers is often reduced during emergencies as stress levels increase, promoting the caregivers' coping capacity is an essential part of fostering good feeding practices for infants and young children
4. The health and vigor of infants and children should be protected so that they are able to suckle frequently and maintain their appetite for complementary foods.
5. Provide support for breastfeeding through assessment of the infant's hydration and nutritional status.
6. Lactating women may be immunized as recommended for adults and adolescents to protect against measles, mumps, rubella, tetanus, diphtheria, pertussis, influenza, Streptococcus pneumonia, Neisseria meningitis, hepatitis A, hepatitis B, varicella, and inactivated polio.
7. Establish a written breastfeeding policy that is routinely comm.-unicated to all healthcare staff.
8. Train all health care staff in skills necessary to implement this policy.
9. Inform all pregnant women about the benefits and management of breastfeeding.
10. Foster the establishment of breastfeeding support groups and refer mothers to them on discharge from the hospital or clinic.

Comply with the International Code

The International Code was the first internationally adopted and endorsed basic minimum requirement to protect healthy practices in respect of infant and young child feeding. Although less binding than a treaty or a convention, the International Code is an international public health recommendation to regulate the marketing of breast milk substitutes, adopted by the World Health Assembly (WHO/UNICEF, 2002). It places the primary obligation on national governments to formulate, implement, monitor, evaluate and adequately fund national policies. The collection of internationally comparable, reliable and valid data on breastfeeding is crucial. Thus the adoption of the WHO guidelines on measurement, monitoring and evaluation of the national situation will be vital (WHO, 2004). Violations of the International Code of Marketing Breast Milk Substitutes (WHO, 1981), and the subsequent relevant WHA Resolutions, which were reaffirmed by all WHO members in 2002, are widespread (Aguayo *et al.,* 2003; IBFAN 2004; IBFAN, 2003; IBFAN, 2001; IBFAN, 1998). Both parents and health professionals are informed by commercial marketing practices (Hawkins and Heard, 2001) and there is evidence that this influences infant feeding decisions (NHMRC,2003; Howard *et al.,* 2003; Perez-Escarmilla *et al.,*1994). Enforcement of the International Code can result in higher levels of breastfeeding (, 2003; Howard *et al.,* 2000; Bradley and Meme, 1992; Rea, 1990; Rea and Berquo, 1990), particularly in the context of multiple approaches to breastfeeding promotion. Specific supports for working mothers, such as the provision of lactation breaks and facilities, can increase breastfeeding rates and duration (McIntyre *et al.,*2002; Valdes *et al.,* 2000; Elgueta *et al.,* 1998). Women anticipating an early return to paid employment report that this influences their decision about whether to initiate or continue breastfeeding (Stewart-Knox *et al.,* 2003; Hamlyn *et al.,* 2002; Netshandama, 2002; NWHB, 2001), thus maternity protection legislation can play a vital role in the decision-making process.

In emergency and relief situations it is important that, as far as possible, infants and young children are breastfed. Artificial feeding in these conditions is difficult and hazardous and leads to increased infant mortality rates (WHO/UNICEF, 2002; IBFAN, 2001). Overseas aid priorities should ensure compliance with internationally recognized best practice guidelines and directives (Jackobsen *et al.,* 2003; WHO, 2003; WHO/UNICEF, 1997). All policies made should be supported by appropriate infrastructural support, and an integrated plan including built-in monitoring and evaluation processes (EU Project, 2004b; Cattaneo and Bussetti, 2001;Hogan, 2001; Bradley, 1992; Rea and Berquo, 1990).

Role of the Relief Agencies

International Lactation Consultant Association (ILCA 1997) has proposed certain guidelines to ensue successful breastfeeding practices during emergencies. These are:

1. Advocate for breastfeeding promotion, protection and support with relief agencies and workers. Infant feeding practices and resources should be assessed, coordinated, and monitored throughout the disaster.

2. Humanitarian aid agencies adopt as part of their policy the promotion and support of breastfeeding in emergency situations. Training humanitarian aid workers to implement these policies is vital as many of them come from non-breastfeeding cultures where basic breastfeeding information and skills are lacking.

3. Training of all humanitarian aid workers include essential breastfeeding messages:

    (a) Nearly every woman can breastfeed her baby (babies) ¨ Mother's milk alone has everything a baby needs to grow well in the first six months of life ¨ Breastfeeding is protective against infectious diseases, especially diarrhea and acute respiratory infections (ARI) ¨ Even malnourished and traumatized mothers produce adequate quantities of good quality milk. The hormones released by the mother in the course of breastfeeding help the mother relax and counteract some of the results of stress.

    (b) When breastfeeding has been stopped prematurely or has not gotten started, re-lactation is possible with adequate support and appropriate breastfeeding management. Inducing lactation in women willing to breastfeed orphaned infants may also be an appropriate strategy. The baby may need supplementary feeding during the transition and families of re-lactating mothers may need help to help the mothers - especially in cultures in which breastfeeding is not widespread.

4. At least one member of each humanitarian team has sufficient breastfeeding management skills to help mothers:

    (a) position and attach their babies to the breast effectively

    (b) inform both mothers and aid workers of the importance of:

    - Keeping mothers and babies together (on average for 8-2 in 24 hours) breastfeeding,
    - co-sleeping and breastfeeding at night,
    - exclusive breastfeeding (no supplements, not even water, tea or breast-milk substitutes) for six months,
    - avoiding the use of artificial teats, dummies and nipple shields

- teach them how to express their milk and feed by cup should the baby be unable to suckle
- teach mothers to introduce others liquids in the second half of the first year with a cup rather than a bottle, while continuing breastfeeding.

5. At least one member of each regional humanitarian team have a high level of lactation management and counseling competency and offer both on-site assessments of non-routine breastfeeding situations and on-going training to upgrade local staff skills. These specialists may be lactation consultants or other health-care professionals with advanced training in lactation and counseling.

6. international and humanitarian aid agencies implement their policies (or develop them in cases where they do not yet have them) to exclude improper donations of breast-milk substitutes and equipment for bottle-feeding, to ensure that any necessary breast-milk substitutes be supplied in quantities sufficient to feed the recipient babies as long as they need them, that these breast-milk substitutes carry generic (non-brand-name) labels and be made available only to those families in which it is documented that there is no possibility for the infants to be breastfed or, during relactation and induced lactation while supplementation is still necessary.

7. Breastfeeding be integrated in national emergency plans in all countries.

8. Public relations and media policies at local, regional, national and international levels emphasize breastfeeding as a vital component in infant health and survival programs during emergencies. There should be a mechanism for quick reaction when media reports imply that emergencies compromise a mother's ability to breastfeed her baby.

9. Donors should be helped to ensure that their donations adhere to the terms of the International Code of Marketing of Breast-milk Substitutes.

RECOMMENDATIONS

Relactation (WHO, 1998)

Support of the mother-baby pair, motivation of the mother and her family and frequent suckling are required for relactation. If the child is still breastfeeding sometimes, breast-milk supply should increase in a few days. If the child has stopped breastfeeding completely, relactation may take 1-2 weeks or more before much breast milk is produced.

1. Develop the motivation of the mother by explaining the importance of breastfeeding and the dangers of formula feeding, especially in emergency situations when access to breast-milk substitutes may not be assure and where the risk of disease and poor access to water and sanitation make feeding with breast-milk substitutes very risky.
2. Support the mother by advising her how to relactate, by supporting her emotionally, by providing her with extra food, water and rest and creating a quiet and private place for breastfeeding.
3. Encourage the mother to keep the child with her as much as possible and to have frequent skin-to-skin content. It is preferable for mother and baby to sleep together.
4. Advise the mother to encourage the baby to suckle as often as possible and whenever he/she appears interested. The baby should suckle ever 1-2 hours, at least 8-12 times within a 24 hour period. The baby should suckle from both breasts. In particular encourage the baby to breastfeed at night.

Breast Milk Substitutes (BMS) (WHO/UNICEF, 2002)

1. Donations of breast milk substitutes (BMS), bottles, teats and commercial baby foods should be refused.
2. If needed, breast milk substitutes should be purchased by the organizations responsible for the nutrition programs, based on a careful analysis and assessment of the situation at hand, and only after approval and together with the appointed emergency health/nutrition

coordinating body and the most senior health/nutrition advisor at headquarters level.

3. Purchased breast milk substitutes should preferably be generically labeled (contact the local UNICEF office about obtaining generically labeled formula).

4. If breast milk substitutes are distributed, their distribution and use should be carefully monitored and infant health followed up by trained health staff. Distribution should only be to infants with a clearly identified need, and for as long as the infants need them (until maximum 1 year age or until breastfeeding is re-established).

5. Breast milk substitutes should NEVER be part of a general distribution.

6. Products should be labeled in accordance with the International Code using correct language, instructions and messages, should comply with the standards Codex Alimentarius, and have a shelf life of at least one year from the date of distribution.

Other Recommendations

1. Every effort should be made to identify ways to breastfeed infants and young children whose mothers are absent or incapacitated, for example by a wet-nurse or through relactation. Those who are responsible for the care of mothers and children should be adequately informed and skilled to support them in breastfeeding (WHO/ UNICEF, 2002).

2. Help from partners, maternal grandmothers and the whole family at large should be sought for informing decisions and supporting breastfeeding mothers (HPA, 2004; Earle, 2002; Hamlyn et al., 2002; Ellis and Waterford Community Care, 2001; Duggan-Jackson, 2000). In particular adequately informed fathers are more likely to encourage and respect breastfeeding and offer appropriate support as required (Stockley, 2004; Arora et al., 2000; Duggan-Jackson, 2000).

3. Intensive support, spanning both the pre- and post-natal periods, have been identified as most effective (Susin et al., 1999;Tedstoneet al., 1998) and can be provided by both health care staff and lay support networks,(e.g. LLL and Cuidiú-ICT), preferably in an integrated manner (Martens, 2002; Pugh et al., 2002).

4. Relatively simple interventions may produce significant increases in breastfeeding rates (Loh *et al.*, 1997), and successful interventions can be located in primary care, hospital or community settings (EU Project, 2004b; Fairbank *et al.*, 2000), but barriers to service provision must be addressed (McCormack, 2003).

5. Evidence based clinical guidelines on the management of breastfeeding need to be agreed and implemented (Renfrew *et al.*, 2000).

6. Numerous studies indicate that current pre-service education for health professionals is rarely sufficient for them to adequately support breastfeeding (Dhandapany et al , 2008; Finneran and Murphy, 2004; Blaauw, 2000; Eden *et al.*, 2000) and there is evidence of a desire for more training (Finneran and Murphy, 2004; Duggan-Jackson, 2000). Strong evidence for the effectiveness of in-service interventions is available (Hillenbrand andLarsen, 2002; Haughwout *et al.*, 2000), particularly for the WHO/UNICEF courses on breastfeeding management and counseling (Kramer *et al.*, 2004; Cattaneo and Buzzetti, 2001; Moran *et al.*, 2000). Substantial evidence exists for their effectiveness in increasing knowledge, skills, initiation and duration of breastfeeding (Su *et al.*, 2007; Labarare *et al.*, 2005; Broadfoot *et al.*, 2005; Kramer *et al.*, 2004; Dulon *et al.*, 2003; Kramer *et al.*, 2003; Kersting and Dulon, 2002; Cattaneo and Buzzetti, 2001; Di Girolamo *et al.*, 2001; Philipp *et al.*, 2001;Radford, 2001; Tappin *et al.*, 2001).

7. Breastfeeding is supported primarily by family and friendship networks (Hamlyn *et al.*, 2002; Fennessy, 1999) and can be threatened by lack of accessible services (WHC, 2002). Community support for breastfeeding can be improved using targeted and localized media and through the availability of local support (Fairbank *et al.*, 2000; Stockley, 2004).

8. Support provided by volunteer mothers is crucial for breastfeeding and is included in one of the ten steps to successful breastfeeding (WHO/UNICEF, 1989).

9. Peer support programmes, such as those provided by LLL, Cuidiú–ICT and support groups facilitated by Public Health Nurses have been found to be valued by mothers (Goonan, 2004; Kyne-Doyle, 2004; Dennis *et al.*, 2002; McInnes and Stone, 2001). When delivered by trained peers or counselors, these programmes have been shown to improve breastfeeding rates (HPA, 2003; Dennis *et al.*, 2002;

Martens, 2002; Pugh *et al.*, 2002; Fairbank *et al.*, 2000; Haider *et al.*, 2000; McInnes *et al.*, 2000).

10. Breastfeeding rates have an inverse relationship with social status; women at most risk of poverty are least likely to initiate and continue breastfeeding (Ward *et al.*, 2004; Gavin, 2002; Twomey *et al.*, 2000). Women experiencing or at risk of social and health inequalities may require specific supports and these necessitate further detailed attention.

11. Women anticipate and experience negative reactions to public breastfeeding (Baker *et al.*, 2003; Greene *et al.*, 2003; Stewart-Knox, B. *et al.*, 2003), which in turn influence their decision-making about infant feeding (Duggan-Jackson, 2000). Thus, the social environment is one crucial target of a comprehensive policy for breastfeeding promotion. Public and commercials places can be rendered breastfeeding friendly with consequent positive outcomes for feeding practices (Mayor, 2004).

12. In long term emergencies, the woman's employment status should be considered. Women frequently report that employment practices influence their decisions about breastfeeding (Greiner, 1999). There are a range of appropriate and effective practices for the support of breastfeeding among workers (McIntyre *et al.*, 2002; Rea *et al.*, 1997) and these can be identified and negotiated between employers and workers (Libbus and Bullock, 2002; Brown *et al.*, 2001; Zinn, 2000; Rea *et al.*, 1999).

13. Media representations of breastfeeding influence decisions to initiate and continue breastfeeding (Stockley, 2004;Earle, 2002; Fairbank *et al.*, 2000), as do perceptions of the appreciation of motherhood by society. Current media representations tend to show artificial feeding more often than breastfeeding and present breastfeeding as more negative and problematic (Henderson *et al.*, 2000). Evidence suggests that localized and targeted media campaigns are more likely to result in increased levels of breastfeeding (Stockley, 2004; Fairbank*et al.*, 2000), while national campaigns are considered effective in awareness raising among decision-makers (EU Project, 2004b).

14. Mothers should be prepared well in advance for emergency situations to appreciate the importance of breastfeeding. The inclusion of breastfeeding education in the curriculum before the statutory school leaving age will help ensure that all potential parents have access to

appropriate information before pregnancy (Campbell and Jones, 1996).

15. Educational interventions should help counteract negative attitudes and perceived practical difficulties associated with breastfeeding (Connolly *et al.,* 1998), but should also positively influence societal perspectives. This will require changes to teacher training curricula (FSAI, 1999) and could usefully include direct contact between young people and nursing mothers (Greene *et al.,* 2003), but evidence suggests that schools require assistance in developing curricular materials (Lockey and Hart, 2003).

SUMMARY

Protecting, promoting and supporting exclusive breastfeeding in emergency situations is particularly important because the risks of illness are higher during emergencies. Breast-milk substitutes carry risks of increased illness and mortality in the best of circumstances, where there is poor hygiene; lack of access to clean water; uncertain supplies of substitutes etc. Reunion of the mother and the child is very important. The initiation of breastfeeding within the first hour of birth and to ensure exclusive breastfeeding for the first six months, is vital. It should also be ensured to start the complementary feeding from six months. Women and their families need extra support and assistance to breastfeed optimally during emergencies. The support that should be provided include 1) counseling and emotional support, 2) practical support in relactation, lactation management, problem solving, positioning etc, 3) quiet and private spaces, 4) extra food and drink for lactating mothers, and 5) avoidance of the use of powdered milks or other breast-milk substitutes. Many myths abound about breastfeeding in emergencies that can undermine both a mother's confidence and the support that she receives   There are some situations when breastfeeding is not possible. These include 1) orphans who have lost their mothers, and where wet-nursing is not possible or acceptable, 2) children temporarily or permanently separated from their mothers, 3) mothers who are very sick and 4) when mothers have stopped breastfeeding for some time and relactation efforts have failed. In these situations the most appropriate food is high quality breast-milk substitutes (BMS) prepared under hygienic conditions, and stored and given safely. BMS or other powdered milks should never be part of a general distribution. They should only be used when breastfeeding is not possible. Clear assessments of the numbers of infants needing BMS should be quickly established in order to ensure adequate supplies and no over-supply. All BMS provided should be labeled in accordance with the International Code of Marketing of Breast-milk Substitutes. In addition, BMS should be provided to caregivers who need it through a separate distribution channel to that of other food aid and be under the close supervision of a trained health worker. Systems should be in place to ensure the use of BMS only by those who need it and to prevent it from 'spilling over' to breastfeeding mother-baby pairs. Moreover, practical and educational support should be provided to ensure BMS. Also, BMS or other powdered milks should never be accepted as donations. The health team and relief workers should have enough skill and awareness regarding the biological and economical benefits of breastfeeding. They should be able to communicate and advocate the practice of breastfeeding effectively. There is a need to work to get agreement between outside agencies and local health workers on breastfeeding policy and practice. They should share up-to-date information on breastfeeding with those who do not have all the facts. Establish mechanisms to ensure that all of the following actions are implemented in a coordinated way. Make sure that maternity care practices follow the WHO/ UNICEF guidelines. Educate the whole community about the benefits of breastfeeding. Highlight the importance of family and social support for breastfeeding. Offer one-to-one assistance for mothers who experience difficulties with breastfeeding. This can be done by helping local women to set up a network through which new mothers can pet practical advice and moral support from other mothers who have successfully breastfed. Another option is to train women to work as breastfeeding counselors. In either case. those who provide support must be sensitive to the culture, health beliefs and circumstances of the mothers they assist. Provide assistance with relactation to mothers of infants who have stopped breastfeeding early.

ACKNOWLEDGMENTS

The first author, in particular, is very much thankful to DAAD (The German Academic Exchange Service) for its support to his PhD studies durig which this work was also completed.

REFERENCES

Aguayo, V.M. Ross, J.S. Kanon, S. and Ouedraogo, A.N. (2003). Monitoring compliance with the International Code of Marketing of Breastmilk Substitutes in west Africa: multisite cross sectional survey in Togo and Burkina Faso. *BMJ,* 326:127–130.

American Academy of Pediatrics, Work Group on Breastfeeding. (1997). Breastfeeding and the use of human milk. *Pediatrics,* 100 (6), 1035-39.

American academy of pediatrics. (2004). Pediatric Nutrition Handbook. 5th ED. American Academy of Pediatrics, 141 Northwest Point Blvd., Elk Grove Village, Il, 847-434-4000.

Arenz, S. Ruckerl, R. Koletzko, B. and von Kries, R. (2004). Breast-feeding and childhood obesity – a systematic review. *Int. J. Obes Relat. Metab. Disord*, 28, 1247–1256.

Arora, S., McJunkin, C., Wehrer, J. and Kuhn, P. (2000). Major factors influencing breastfeeding rates: Mothers perception of father's attitude and milk supply. *Pediatrics,* 106, 1126.

Ascherio, A., Chase, R., Cote T., Dehaes, G., Hoskins, E., Laaouej, J. and *et al.* (1992). Effect of the Gulf War on infant and child mortality in Iraq. *N. Engl. J. Med.*, 327, 931-6.

Bachrach, V.R. Schwarz, E. and Bachrach, L.R. (2003). Breastfeeding and the risk of hospitalization for respiratory disease in infancy: a meta-analysis. *Arch. Pediatr. Adolesc. Med,* 157, 237-43.

Baker, L., Lavender, T. and McFadden, K. (2003) Family Life and Breastfeeding, In Department of Health, Infant Feeding Initiative – A Report Evaluating the Breastfeeding Practice Projects 1999-2002. Department of Health: London.

Ball, T.M. and Wright, A. (1999). Health care costs of formula feeding in the first year of life. *Pediatrics*, 103, 870- 876.

Barr, R.G. and Menzies, R. (1994). The effect of war on tuberculosis: Results of a tuberculin survey among displaced persons in El Salvador and a review of the literature. *Tuber Lung Dis.,* 75, 251-9.

Blaauw, M. (2000). A closer look at breastfeeding in medical handbooks and teaching material in the Netherlands. Vrije Universiteit, Amsterdam / Institute of Public Health: Copenhagen.

Black, R.E. Morris, S. S. and Bryce J. (2003). Where and why are 10 million children dying every year? *Lancet,* 361, 2226-34.

Bloland, P.B. Williams, H.A. (2003). Malaria control during mass population movements and natural disasters. Washington (DC): The National Academies Press.

Bradley, J.E. and Meme, J. (1992). Breastfeeding promotion in Kenya: changes in health worker knowledge, attitudes and practices, 1982-89. *Journal of Tropical Pediatrics*, 38, 228-34.

Breastfeeding in Ireland. (2005). *A five-year strategic action plan National Committee on Breastfeeding*. Department of Health and Children, Ireland.

Breastfeeding Promotion Network of India (BPNI). 2005. Infant Feeding in Emergency Situations: A report from the National Convention of BPNI Breastfeeding Promotion Network of India (BPNI), BP-3, Pitampura Delhi 110034, pp-5.

Broadfoot, M. and Britten, J., Tappin, D.M. and MacKenzie, J.M. (2005). The Baby Friendly Hospital Initiative and breastfeeding rates in Scotland. *Archives of Disease in Childhood Fetal and Neonatal*. 90, F114-F116.

Brown, C.A., Poag, S. and Kasprzycki, C. (2001). Exploring large employers' and small employers' knowledge, attitudes, and practices on breastfeeding support in the workplace. *Journal of Human Lactation*, 17, 39-46.

Campbell, H. and Jones, I.G. (1996). Promoting breastfeeding: a view of the current position and a proposed agenda for action in Scotland. *Journal of Public Health Medicine*, 18, 406- 414.

Cattaneo, A. and Buzzetti, R. (2001). Effect on rates of breast feeding of training for the baby friendly hospital initiative. *British Medical Journal*, 323, 1358-62.

Cattaneo, A. and Buzzetti, R. (2001). Effect on rates of breast feeding of training for the baby friendly hospital initiative. *British Medical Journal*, 323, 1358-62.

Cattaneo, A. Ronfani, L. Burmaz, T. Quintero-Romero, S. Macaluso, A. and Di Mario, S. (2006). Infant feeding and cost of health care: a cohort study. *Acta Paediatr*, 2006; 95: 540-546.

CDC. Centers for Disease Control. (1992). Famine-affected, refugee, and displaced populations: recommendations for public health issues. U.S. Department of Health and Human Services Public Health Service Centers for Disease Control Atlanta, Georgia 30333. MMWR, 41, (No. RR-13), 1-76.

Chen A, Rogan WJ. (2004). Breastfeeding and the risk of postneonatal death in the United States. *Pediatrics*, 113, e435-e439.

Chung, M. Raman, R. Trikalinos, T. Lau, J. and Ip, S. (2008). Interventions in Primary Care to Promote Breastfeeding: An Evidence Review for the U.S. Preventive Services Task Force. *Ann. of Intern. Med.,* 149. 565-582.

Cohen, R.J. Brown, K.H. Canahuati, J. Rivera, L.L. and Dewey, K.G. (1995). Determinants of growth from birth to 12 months among breastfed Honduran infants in relation to age of introduction of complementary foods. *Pediatrics* 96(3), 504–510.

Connolly, C. Kelleher, C.C. Becker, G. Friel, S. and Nic Gabhainn, S. (1998). Attitudes of young men and women to breastfeeding. *Irish Medical Journal*, (3), 88-89.

Cunningham, A.S. Jelliffe, D.B. and Jelliffe, E.F.P. (1991). Breastfeeding and health in the 1980s: A global epidemiologic review. *Journal of Pediatrics*, 118 (5), 659 -666.

Cunningham, A.S. (1995). Breastfeeding: Adaptive behavior for child health and longevity. In P. Stuart-Macadam and K.A. Dettwyler (Eds.) *Breastfeeding: Biocultural Perspectives*. New York: Walter de Gruyter.

Daly, S.E. and Hartmann, P.E. (1995). Infant demand and milk supply. Part 1: Infant demand and milk production in lactating women. *Journal of Human Lactation*, 11(1), 21–6.

Dennis, C.L., Hodnett, E., Gallop, R. and Chalmers, B. (2002). The effect of peer support on breast-feeding duration among primiparous women: a randomized controlled trial. *Canadian Medical Association Journal*, 166, 21-8.

Dennis, C.L., Hodnett, E., Gallop, R. and Chalmers, B. (2002). The effect of peer support on breast- feeding duration among primiparous women: a randomized controlled trial. *Canadian Medical Association Journal*, 166, 21-8.

Desenclos, J.C. Michel D. Tholly, F. Magdi, I. Pecoul, B. Desve, G. 1990. Mortality trends among refugees in Honduras, 1984-1987. *Int. J. Epidemiol,* 19, 367-73.

DeWald, L. and Fountain, L. (2006). Introducing Emergency Preparedness in Childbirth Education Classes. *J. Perinat., Educ,* 15(1), 49–51.

Dewey, K.G. Heinig, M.J. Nommsen, L.A. Lonnerdal, B. 2001. Adequacy of energy intake among breastfed infants in the DARLING study: Relationships to growth velocity, morbidity, and activity levels. *J. Pediatrics*, 119, 538–547.

Dhandapany, G. Bethou, A. Arunagirinathan, A. and Ananthakrishnan, S. (2008). Antenatal counseling on breastfeeding–is it adequate? A descriptive study from Pondicherry, India *International Breastfeeding Journal*, 3 (5).

Di Girolamo, A.M., Grummer-Strawn, L.M. and Fein, S. (2001). Maternity care practices: implications for breastfeeding. *Birth*, 28, 94-100.

Diane Thulier, D. (2009). Breastfeeding in America: A History of Influencing Factors. *J. Hum. Lact*, 25-96.

DOHC.(2003). *Interim Report of the National Committee on Breastfeeding*. Health Promotion Unit, Department of Health and Children, Dublin.

Dowell, S.F. Toko, A. Sita, C. Piarroux, R. Duerr, A. Woodruff, B.A. (1995). Health and nutrition in centers for unaccompanied refugee children. Experience from the 1994, Rwandan refugee crisis. *JAMA*, 273, 1802-6.

Drane, D. (1997). Breastfeeding and formula feeding: a preliminary economic analysis. *Breastfeeding Review*, 5 (1), 7-15.

Duggan-Jackson, A. (2000). *Breastfeeding: A midland health board perspective*. Department of Public Health, Midland Health Board: Tullamore.

Duggan-Jackson, A. (2000). *Breastfeeding: A midland health board perspective*. Department of Public Health, Midland Health Board: Tullamore.

Dulon, M. Kersting, M. and Bender, R. (2003). Breastfeeding promotion in non-UNICEF- certified hospitals and long-term breastfeeding success in Germany. *Acta Paediatrica*, 92 (6), 653-8.

Duncan, B. Ey J. Holberg, C.J. and *et al.* (1993). Exclusive breast-feeding for at least 4 months protects against otitis media. *Pediatrics*, 91:867.

Earle, S. (2002). Factors affecting the initiation of breastfeeding: implications for breastfeeding promotion. *Health Promotion International*, 17 (3), 205-214.

Eden, A.N., Mir, M.A. and Srinivasan, P. (2000). The pediatric forum: breastfeeding education of pediatric residents: A national survey. *Archives of Pediatric and Adolescent Medicine*, 154, 1271-2.

Ellis, A. and Waterford Community Care. (2001). *Promotion of breastfeeding Pilot Project Report*. South Eastern Health Board, Ireland.

EU Project on Promotion of Breastfeeding in Europe .(2004). Protection, promotion and support of breastfeeding in Europe: review of interventions. European Commission, Directorate Public Health and Risk Assessment, Luxembourg. http://europa.eu.int/comm/health/ph_pr ojects/2002/promotion/promotion_2002_18_en.htm.

EU Project on Promotion of Breastfeeding in Europe. (2004). Protection, promotion and support of breastfeeding in Europe: review of interventions. European Commission, Directorate Public Health and Risk Assessment, Luxembourg.

Fairbank, L., O'Meara, S., Renfrew, M.J., Woolridge, M., Sowden, A.J. and Lister-Sharp, D. (2000). A systematic review to evaluate the effectiveness of interventions to promote the initiation of breastfeeding. *Health Technology Assessment*, 4 (25), 1-171.

Finneran, B. and Murphy, K. (2004). Breast is best for GPs—or is it? Breastfeeding attitudes and practice of general practitioners in the Mid-West of Ireland. *Irish Medical Journal*, 97 (9), 268-270.

FSAI. (1999). *Recommendations for a National Infant Feeding Policy*. Food Safety Authority of Ireland: Dublin.

Gavin, B. (2002). A report on the pilot project to promote breastfeeding in community care area 1 and recommendations to promote and support breastfeeding in the Area Health Boards. Department of Health Promotion, East Coast Area Health Board and Breastfeeding Support Committee Community Care Area 1, Dublin.

Goldman, A.S. Chheda, S. Keeney, S.E. and *et al.* (1994). Immunologic protection of the premature newborn by human milk. *Semin. Perinatol* 1994; 18:495.

Goonan, N. (2004). *Breastfeeding Support Groups*. Unpublished MA thesis, Department of Health Promotion, NUI Galway.

Greco, L. Auricchio, S. Mayer, M. And *et al.* (1988). Case control study on nutritional risk factors in celiac disease. *J. Pediatr. Gastroenterol. Nutr.* 1988,7:395–9.

Greene, J., Stewart-Knox, B. and Wright, M. (2003). Feeding preferences and attitudes to breastfeeding and its promotion among teenagers in Northern Ireland. *Journal of Human Lactation,* 19 (1), 57-65.

Greiner, T. (1999). Factors associated with the duration of breastfeeding may depend on the extent to which mothers of young children are employed. *Acta Paediatrica*, 88, 1311-1312

Haider, R., Ashworth, A., Kabir, I. and Huttly, S.R. (2000). Effect of community-based peer counsellors on exclusive breastfeeding practices in Dhaka, Bangladesh: a randomised controlled trial. *Lancet*, 356, 1643-1647.

Hamlyn, B. Brooker, S. Oleinikova, K. and Wands, S. (2002). *Infant Feeding 2000*. Office for National Statistics, The Stationary Office: London.

Hamlyn, B. Brooker, S. Oleinikova, K. and *et al.* (2002). *Infant feeding 2000*. A survey conducted on behalf of UK Health Departments by BMRB Social Research. The Stationery Office, London.

Haughwout, J.C., Eglash, A.R., Plane, M.B., Mundt, M.P. and Fleming, M.F. (2000). Improving residents' breastfeeding assessment skills: a problem-based workshop. *Family Practice,* 17, 541-6.

Heinig M.J. (2005). Hope in the Darkest Days: Breastfeeding Support in Emergencies. *J. Hum. Lact*, 21, 395.

Henderson, L., Kitzinger, J. and Green, J. (2000). Representing infant feeding: content analysis of British media portrayals of bottle-feeding and breast-feeding. *British Medical Journal*, 321,1196-8.

Hill, P.D., Aldag, J.C. Chatterton, R. T. and Zinaman, M. (2005). Primary and Secondary Mediators' Influence on Milk Output in Lactating Mothers of Preterm and Term Infants, *J. Hum. Lact*, 21(2), 138 - 150.

Hillenbrand, K.M. and Larsen, P.G. (2002). Effect of an educational intervention about breastfeeding on the knowledge, confidence, and behaviors of pediatric resident physicians. *Pediatrics,* 110, e59.

Hogan, S.E. (2001) Overcoming barriers to breastfeeding: suggested breastfeeding promotion programs for communities in eastern Nova Scotia. *Canadian Journal of Public Health*, 92, 105-8.

Horta B.L. Bahl, R. Martines, J. and Victora, C. (2007). *Evidence on the long-term effects of breastfeeding: systematic reviews and meta-analyses.* Geneva: World Health Organization.

Howard C, Howard F, Lawrence R, Andresen E, DeBlieck E, Weitzman M. (2000). prenatal formula advertising and its effect on breast-feeding patterns. *Obstet. Gynecol*, 95(2), 296-303.

Howard, C.R. Howard, F.M. Lanphear, B. Eberly, S. de Blieck, E.A., Oakes, D. and *et al.* (2003). Randomized clinical trial of pacifier use and bottle-feeding or cup feeding and their effect on breastfeeding. *Pediatrics*, 111, 511-8.

HPA. (2003). Peer support as an intervention to increase the incidence and duration of breastfeeding in Northern Ireland: what is the evidence? Belfast: Health Promotion Agency for Northern Ireland.

HPA. (2003). Peer support as an intervention to increase the incidence and duration of breastfeeding in Northern Ireland: what is the evidence? Belfast: Health Promotion Agency for Northern Ireland.

Hyman, S. and Stanner, S. (2004). Facts Behind The Headlines: Dispelling popular myths that discourage breastfeeding. *Nutrition Bulletin*, 29 (3), 180-3.

IBFAN Asia / Breastfeeding Promotion Network of India (BPNI) and UNICEF ROSA organized "Infant Feeding and HIV: A Regional

Colloquium for the Asia Pacific" held on 28-29 November 2003, New Delhi, India.

IBFAN. (2001). Breaking the rules, stretching the rules: Evidence of Violations of the International Code of Marketing of Breast-milk Substitutes and subsequent Resolutions. *A report by International Baby Food Action Network (IBFAN)*, Published by IBFAN, S/B P.O. Box 19, 10700 Penang, Malaysia, 25-31.

IBFAN. (2003). Using international tools to stop corporate malpractice: does it work? International Baby Food Action Network, Cambridge (http://www .ibfan.org/english/pdfs/casestudies04.pdf.)

IBFAN.(2004). How breastfeeding is undermined. International Baby Food Action Network,(www.ibreastfeedingan.org/english/issue/breastfe.html.)

Infant feeding in emergencies. (1997). A guide for mothers. Prepared for the Program for Nutrition Policy, Infant Feeding and Food Security. Lifestyles and Health Unit World Health Organization Regional Office for Europe, Copenhagen.

Infant Feeding in Emergency Situations. (2005). *A report from the National Convention of BPNI*. Breastfeeding Promotion Network of India (BPNI), BP-33Pitampura, Delhi 110 034.

Institute of Medicine. (1991). *Nutrition during lactation*. Washington, DC: National Academy Press.

International Lactation Consultant Association (ILCA). Position on infant feeding in emergencies. ILCA, 2501 Aerial Center Parkway · Suite 103 Morrisville, NC 27560 USA.

Ip S, Chung M, Raman G, Chew P, Magula N, DeVine D, *et al.* (2007). Breastfeeding and maternal and infant health outcomes in developed countries. Evidence Report/Technology Assessment No. 153. Rockville, MD: Agency for Healthcare Research and Quality.

Jakobsen, M.S. Sodemann, M. Mølbak, K. Alvarenga, I.J. Nielsen, J. Aaby, P. (2003). Termination of breastfeeding after 12 months of age due to a new pregnancy and other causes is associated with increased mortality in Guinea-Bissau. *Int. J. Epidemiol.*, 32, 92–96.

Jones, G. Steketee, R.W. Black, R.E. Bhutta, Z.A. Morris, S.S. (2003). How many child deaths can we prevent this year? *Lancet*, 362, 65-71.

Katona-Apte, J. and Mokdad, A. (1998). Malnutrition of children in the Democratic People's Republic of North Korea. *J. Nutr.*, 128, 1315-9.

Kawasaki, M.P. (2005). M*othering with Breastfeeding and Maternal Care: Breastfeeding myths*. Ist. Ed. iUniverse Publishers, iUniverse, Inc., 1663 Liberty Drive, Suite 300, Bloomington, IN 47403, pp. 102-200.

Kawasaki, M.P. (2005). *Mothering with Breastfeeding and Maternal Care: Breastfeeding myths*. Ist. Ed. iUniverse Publishers, iUniverse, Inc., 1663 Liberty Drive, Suite 300, Bloomington, IN 47403, pp. 102-200.

Kelly M. (1993). Infant feeding in emergencies. *Disasters,* 17 (2), 110–121.

Kersting, M. and Dulon, M. (2002) Assessment of breast- feeding promotion in hospitals and follow-up survey of mother-infant pairs in Germany: the SuSe Study. *Public Health Nutrition*, 5, 547-552.

Khan, M.U. Munshi, M.H. (1983). Clinical illness and causes of death in a Burmese refugee camp in Bangladesh. Int J Epidemiol, 12, 460-4.

Klement, E. Cohen, R.V. Boxman, A. Joseph, and Reif, S. (2004). Breastfeeding and risk of inflammatory bowel disease: a systematic review with meta-analysis. *Am. J. Clinical Nutrition*, 80(5), 1342-52.

Kramer, M.S., Guo, T., Platt, R.W., Sevkovskaya, Z., Dzikovich, I., Collet, J.P., Shapiro, S., Chalmers, B., Hodnett, E., Vanilovich, I., Mezen, I., Ducruet, T., Shishko, G. and Bogdanovich, N. (2003). Infant growth and health outcomes associated with 3 compared with 6 mo ofexclusive breastfeeding. *American Journal of Clinical Nutrition*, 78, 291-295.

Kramer, M.S., Kakuma, R. (2004). The optimal duration of exclusive breastfeeding. A systematic review. *Adv. Exp. Med. Biol.*, 554:63-77.

Kull I. Wickman, M. Lilja, G. Nordvall, S.L. and Pershagen, G. (2002). Breast feeding and allergic diseases in infants--a prospective birth cohort study. *Arch. Dis. Child*, 87, 478-481.

Kull, I. Almqvist, C. Lilja, G. Pershagen, G. and Wickman, M. (2004). Breast-feeding reduces the risk of asthma during the first 4 years of life. *J. Allergy Clin. Immunol.*, 114, 755-60.

Kwan, M.L. Buffler, P.A. Abrams, B. And Kiley, V.A. (2004). Breastfeeding and the risk of childhood leukemia: a meta-analysis. *Public Health Rep*, 19, 521-35.

Kyne-Doyle, M. (2004). *Consumer Satisfaction Survey of Breast Feeding Support Groups/clinics*, Community Care Area 1, ECAHB: Dublin

La Leche League. (2006). Answers Questions about Breastfeeding in Emergencies. La Leche League International (LLLI), Schaumburg, IL 60168-4079, USA (available on: http://www.lalecheleague.org/em ergencyfaq.html)

Labarere J, Gelbert-Baudino N, Ayral AS, Duc C, Berchotteau M, Bouchon N, Schelstraete C, Vittoz JP, Francois P, Pons JC. (2005). Efficacy of breastfeeding support provided by trained clinicians during an early, routine, preventive visit: a prospective, randomized, open trial of 226 mother-infant pairs. *Pediatrics*, 115(2), 139-46.

Libbus, M.K. and Bullock, L.F. (2002). Breastfeeding and employment: an assessment of employer attitudes. *Journal of Human Lactation*, 18, 247-51.

Lin SS, Chien LY, Tai CJ, Lee CF: Effectiveness of a prenatal education programme on breastfeeding outcomes in Taiwan. *J. Clin. Nurs*, in press.

Lockey, R. and Hart, A. (2003). Addressing inequalities in health: The Breast Benefits project. *British Journal of Midwifery*, 11 (5), 281-287.

Loh, N.R. Kelleher, C.C. Long, S. and Loftus, BG. (1997). Can we increase breastfeeding rates? *Irish Medical Journal*, 90 (3), 100-101.

Lois B. Dusdieker, Phyllis J. Stumbo, Brenda M. Booth, Rosemary N. and Wilmoth, M.A. (1990). Prolonged Maternal Fluid Supplementation in Breast-Feeding. *Pediatrics,* 86 (5), 737-740

Marild, S. Hansson, S. Jodal, U. Oden, A. and Svedberg, K. (2004). Protective effect of breastfeeding against urinary tract infection. *Acta Paediatr*, 93(2), 154-6.

Martens, P.J. (2002). Increasing breastfeeding initiation and duration at a community level: an evaluation of Sagkeeng First Nation's community health nurse and peer counselor programs. *Journal of Human Lactation*, 18, 236-46.

Mason, J.B. (2002). Lessons on nutrition of displaced people. *J. Nutr.*, 132, 2096S-103S.

Mayor, S. (2004). Report warns of continuing violations of code on breast milk. British *Medical Journal*, 328, 1218.

McCormack, A. (2003). *An audit of the breastfeeding service in community care area* 8. Northern Area Health Board: Dublin.

McInnes, R.J. and Stone, D.H. (2001). The process of implementing a community-based peer breast- feeding support programme: the Glasgow experience. *Journal of Public Health Medicine,* 22 (2), 138-145.

McInnes, R.J., Love, J.G. and Stone, D.H. (2000). Evaluation of a community-based intervention to increase breastfeeding prevalence. *Journal of Public Health Medicine*, 22, 138-145.

McIntyre, E. Pisaniello, D. Gun, R., Sanders, C. and Frith, D. (2002). Balancing breastfeeding and paid employment: a project targeting employers, women and workplaces. *Health Promotion International*, 17 (3), 215-22.

McIntyre, E. Pisaniello,D. Gun, D. Sanders, C. and Frith, D. (2002). Balancing breastfeeding and paid employment: a project targeting employers, women and workplaces. *Health Promotion International*, Vol. 17, No. 3, 215-222, September 2002.

Mead, M.N. (2008). Contaminants in Human Milk-Weighing the Risks against the Benefits of Breastfeeding. *Environmental Health Perspectives*, 116 (10), A426-35.

Meek JY. (2002). *New Mother's Guide to Breastfeeding: American Academy of Pediatrics*. New York, Bantam Books.

Montgomery, D.L. and Splett, P.L. (1997). Economic benefit of breast-feeding infants enrolled in WIC. *Journal of the American Dietetic Association*, 97(4), 379-385

Moran, V.H., Bramwell, R., Dykes, F. and Dinwoodie, K.(2000). An evaluation of skills acquisition on the WHO/UNICEF Breastfeeding Management Course using the pre-validated Breastfeeding Support Skills Tool (BeSST). *Midwifery*, 16, 197- 203.

Mortensen, E.L. Michaelsen, K.F. Sanders, S.A. and Reinisch, J.M. (2002). The association between duration of breastfeeding and adult intelligence. *JAMA*, 8;287(18), 2365-71.

Mortensen, E.L., Michaelsen, K.F. Sanders, S.A. and Reinisch, J.M. (2002). The association between duration of breastfeeding and adult intelligence. *JAMA,* 287, 2365–2371.

Moss, W.J. Ramakrishnan, M. Storms, D. Henderson, A. and *et al.* 2006. Child health in complex emergencies. *Bull. World Health Organ* vol.84 no.1

National Health and Medical Research Council. (2003). Dietary guidelines for children and adolescents in Australia incorporating the infant feeding guidelines for health workers. AusInfo, Canberra.

Netshandama, V.O. (2002). Breastfeeding practices of working women. *Curationis,* 25(1), 21-7.

NWHB. (2001). Breast is Best: Knowing is not enough. Departments of Public Health and HealthPromotion, North-Western Health Board: Manorhamilton.

O'Connor, M.E. Burkle, T.M. Olness, K. (2001). Infant feeding practices in complex emergencies: A. case study approach. *Prehosp. Disast. Med.* 16(4), 231–238.

Oddy, W.H. Kendall, G.E. Blair, E. De Klerk, N.H. Stanley, F.J. Landau, L.I. and *et al.* (2003). Breast feeding and cognitive development in childhood: a prospective birth cohort study. *Paediatr Perinat Epidemiol*, 7, 81-90.

Owen, C.G, Whincup, P.H. Gilg, J.A. and Cook, D.G. (2003). Effect of breast feeding in infancy on blood pressure in later life: systematic review and meta-analysis. *BMJ,* 327, 1189-95

Pabst, H.F. Godel, J. Grace, M. Cho, H. and Spady, D.W. (1989). Effect of breast-feeding on immune response to BCG vaccination. *Lancet,* 11:1(8633), 295–297.

Pelletier, D.L. Frongillo, E.A. Jr. Schroeder, D.G. Habicht, J.P. (1995). The effects of malnutrition on child mortality in developing countries. *Bull. World Health Org.*, 73, 443-8.

Perez-Escamilla, R. Lutter, C. Segall, A.M. and Rivera, A. Trevino-Siller, S. and Sanghvi, T. (1995). Exclusive breast-feeding duration is associated with attitudinal, socioeconomic and biocultural determinants in three Latin American countries. *J. Nutr.,* 125, 2972–84.

Perez-Escamilla, R. Pollitt, E. Leonardo, B. and Dewey, K.G. (1994). Infant feeding policies in maternity wards and their effect on breast-feeding success: an analytical overview. *Am. J. Public Health*, 84, 89–97.

Peterson, E.A. Roberts, L. Toole, M.J. Peterson, D.E. (1998).The effect of soap distribution on diarrhea: Nyamithuthu Refugee Camp. *Int. J. Epidemiol.*, 27, 520-4.

Pettitt, D.J. Forman M.R. Hanson, R.L. Knowler, W.C. Bennett, P.H. (1997). Breastfeeding and incidence of non-insulin-dependent diabetes mellitus in Pima Indians. *Lancet,* 19, 350(9072), 166-8.

Phillip, B.L., Merewood, A., Miller, L.W., Chawla, N., Murphy-Smith, M.M., Gomes, J.S., Cimo, S. and Cook, J.T. (2001). Baby-Friendly Hospital initiative improves breastfeeding initiation rates in a US Hospital Setting. *Pediatrics*, 108, 677- 68.

Porter, J.D. Gastellu-Etchegorry, M. Navarre, I. Lungu, G. and Moren, A. (1990). Measles outbreaks in the Mozambican refugee camps in Malawi: the continued need for an effective vaccine. *Int. J. Epidemiol*, 19, 1072-7.

Prentice, A. M., Paul, A. A. Prentice, A. Black, A. Cole T. and Whitehead R. (1986). Cross-cultural differences in lactational performance. In: Hamosh M, Goldmans AS, eds. *Human lactation 2: Maternal and environmental factors*. New York: Plenum Press, 13-44.

Prentice, A.M. Goldberg, G.R. and Prentice, A. (1994). Body mass index and lactation performance. *Eur. J. Clin. Nutr.,* 48S, 78-89.

Puoane, T. Sanders, D. Chopra, M. and *et al.* (2001). Evaluating the clinical management of severely malnourished children: A study of two rural district hospitals. *The South African Medical Journal*, 91(2), 137–141.

Radford, A. (2001). UNICEF is crucial in promoting and supporting breastfeeding. *British Medical Journal*, 322, 555.

Radford, A. (2002). Breast-feeding campaign could save a fortune. *Health Service Journal*, 112, 27.

Rautava, S. and Walker, W.A. (2009). Academy of Breastfeeding Medicine Founder's Lecture 2008: Breastfeeding—An Extrauterine Link Between Mother and Child. *Breastfeeding Medicine*, 4(1), 3-10.

Rea, M.F. (1990). The Brazilian National Breastfeeding Program: a success story. *International Journal of Gynaecology and Obstetrics*, 31 Suppl 1, 79-82.

Rea, M.F. and Berquo, E.S. (1990) Impact of the Brazilian national breastfeeding program on mothers in greater Sao Paulo. *Bulletin of the World Health Organization*, 68, 365-71.

Renfrew, M.J. Woolridge, M.W. and Ross-McGill, H. (2000). *Enabling women to breastfeed: A structured review with evidence-based guidance for practice*. The Stationary Office: London.

Renfrew, M.J., Woolridge, M.W. and Ross-McGill, H. (2000). *Enabling women to breastfeed: A structured review with evidence-based guidance for practice*. Office for National Statistics, the Stationary Office: London.

Ressler, E.M. Boothby, N. Steinbock, D.J. (1988). *Unaccompanied children: care and protection in wars, natural disasters, and refugee movements*. New York: Oxford University Press.

Rice, A.L. Sacco, L. Hyder, A. and Black, R.E. (2000). Malnutrition as an underlying cause of childhood deaths associated with infectious diseases in developing countries. *Bull., World Health Organ.*, 78, 1207-21.

Riordan, S.J. (1997). The cost of not breastfeeding: A commentary. *Journal of Human Lactation,* 13(2), 93-97.

Roberts, L. Chartier, Y. Chartier, O. Malenga, G. Toole, M. and Rodka, H. (2001). Keeping clean water clean in a Malawi refugee camp: a randomized intervention trial. *Bull World Health Organ.*, 79, 280-7.

Rowland, M. Munir, A. Durrani, N. Noyes ,H. and Reyburn, H. (1999). An outbreak of cutaneous leishmaniasis in an Afghan refugee settlement in north-west Pakistan. *Trans R. Soc. Trop. Med. Hyg.*, 93, 133-6.

RSM. (2000). Effective Health Care: Promoting the initiation of breastfeeding. *Royal Society of Medicine: NHS Centre for Reviews and Dissemination*, University of York.

Santaniello-Newton, A. and Hunter, P.R. (2000). Management of an outbreak of meningococcal meningitis in a Sudanese refugee camp in Northern Uganda. *Epidemiol Infect*, 24, 75-81.

Sapir, D.G. (1993). Natural and man-made disasters: the vulnerability of women-headed households and children without families. *World Health Stat.*, 46, 227-33.

Shears, P. (1991). Epidemiology and infection in famine and disaster. *Epidemiol. Infect,* 107:241-54.

Shears, P. Berry, A.M. Murphy, R. and Nabil, M.A. (1987). Epidemiological assessment of the health and nutrition of Ethiopian refugees in emergency camps in Sudan, 1985. *BMJ* (Clin Res Ed), 295:314-8.

Shu, X.O. Linet, M.S. Steinbuch, M. Wen, W.Q. Buckley, J.D. Neglia, J.P. Potter, J.D. Reaman, G.H. and Robison, L.L. (1999). Breast-feeding and risk of childhood acute leukemia. *J. Natl. Cancer Inst,* 91, 1765–1772.

Siddique, A.K. Salam, A. Islam, M.S. Akram, K. Majumdar, R.N. Zaman, K. and *et al.* (1995). Why treatment centres failed to prevent cholera deaths among Rwandan refugees in Goma, Zaire. *Lancet,* 345, 359-61.

Stephen R. P. and George R. B. (2009). Fertility Awareness-Based Methods: Another Option for Family Planning. *The Journal of the American Board of Family Medicine* 22 (2): 147-157.

Stewart-Knox, B. Gardiner K. and Wright, M. (2003). What is the problem with breast-feeding? A qualitative analysis of infant feeding perceptions. *Journal of Human Nutrition and Dietetics* 16, 265–273.

Stockley, L. (2004). *Consolidation and updating the evidence base for promotion of breastfeeding.* Cardiff, National Health Service, Wales.

Su, L.L. Chong, Y.C. Chan, Y.H. Chan, Y.S. and *et al.* (2007). Antenatal education and postnatal support strategies for improving rates of exclusive breast feeding: randomised controlled trial. *BMJ,* 335, 574-575.

Susin, L.R. Giugliani, E.R. Kummer, S.C. Maciel, M. Simon, C. and da Silveira, L.C. (1999). Does parental breastfeeding knowledge increase breastfeeding rates? B*irth,* 26, 149-56.

Swerdlow, D.L. Malenga, G. Begkoyian, G. Nyangulu, D. Toole, M. Waldman, R.J. and *et al.* (1987). Epidemic cholera among refugees in Malawi, Africa: treatment and transmission. *Epidemiol Infect* 118, 207-14.

Tappin, D.M., Mackenzie, J.M., Brown, A.J., Girdwood, R.W., Britten, J., Broadfoot, M. and Warren, J. (2001). Breastfeeding rates are increasing in Scotland. *Health Bulletin* (Edinb), 59, 102-113.

Tedstone, A.E. Dunce, N. and Aviles, M. (1998). Effectiveness of interventions to promote healthy feeding of infants under one year of age: a review. *Health Education Authority:* London.

Todd, J.M. Parnell, W.R. (1994). Nutrient intakes of women who are breastfeeding. *Eur. J. Clin. Nutr.,* 48(8), 567-74.

Toole, M.J. and Waldman, R.J. (1990). Prevention of excess mortality in refugee and displaced populations in developing countries. *JAMA,* 263, 3296-3302.

Toole, M.J. and Waldman, R.J. (1997). The public health aspects of complex emergencies and refugee situations. *Annu. Rev. Public Health*, 18, 283-312.

Tuttle, C.R. and Dewey, K.G. (1996). Potential cost savings for Medical, AFDC, food stamps and WIC programs associated with increase in breastfeeding among low income among women in California. *Journal of American Dietetic Association*, 96, 885-890.

Twomey, A., Kilberd, B., Matthews, T. and O'Reagan, M. (2000). Feeding infants – an investment in the future. *Irish Medical Journal*, 98, 248-250.

UNICEF/UNHCR. (1994). United Nations Children's Fund/United Nations High Commissioner for Refugees Joint Task Force. *Standards for Protection and Care of Unaccompanied Refugee Children*; Rwanda Refugee Operation, Goma (Zaire). New York: United Nations Children's Fund.

United States Breastfeeding Committee. (2008). Statement on the Safe Use of Donor Human Milk. Washington, DC: United States Breastfeeding Committee, 2025 M Street, NW, Suite 800 Washington DC 20036.

United States Breastfeeding Committee. (2008). S*tatement on the Safe Use of Donor Human Milk.* Washington, DC: United States Breastfeeding Committee, 2025 M Street, NW, Suite 800 Washington DC 20036.

US Department of Health and Human Services. (2000). *Healthy People 2010: Conference Edition.* Volumes I and II. Washington, DC: US Department of Health and Human Services, Office of the Assistant Secretary of Health.

US Dept of Commerce. (1999). Poverty 1998. US Department of Commerce, Census Bureau: Washington DC. www.census.gov/hhe/poverty.

Valdes V, Pugin E, Schooley J, Catalan S, Aravena R. (2000). Clinical support can make the difference in exclusive breastfeeding success among working women. *J. Trop. Pediatr.*, 46(3): 14 - 154.

Valente, F. Otten, M. Balbina, F. Van de, W.R. Chezzi, C. Eriki, P. and *et al.* (2000). Massive outbreak of poliomyelitis caused by type-3 wild poliovirus in Angola in 1999. *Bull. World Health Organ*, 78, 339-46.

Vennemann, M.M. Bajanowski, T. . Brinkmann, B. Jorch, D. Yücesan, K. Sauerland, C. Mitchell, E.A. and the GeSID Study Group. (2009). Does Breastfeeding Reduce the Risk of Sudden Infant Death Syndrome. *Pediatrics,* 123 (3), e406-e410.

Ward, M., Sheridan, A., Howell, F., Hegarty, I. and O'Farrell, A. (2004). Infant feeding: factors affecting initiation, exclusivity and duration. *Irish Medical. Journal*, 97 (7), 197-199.

Webster, B. (2000). Medical and financial cost associated with artificial infant feeding. Annual Conference of the International Lactation Consultant Association 1997. Cited in Northern Ireland Breastfeeding Strategy Group. Breastfeeding Strategy for Northern Ireland. Department of Health and Social Services(DHSS).

Weimer, J.P. (2001). The economic benefits of breastfeeding. *Food Review*, 24 (2), 23-26.

Weise, P.Z. and de Benoist, B. (2002). Meeting the challenges of micronutrient deficiencies in emergency-affected populations. *Proc. Nutr. Soc.*, 61, 251-7.

WHC. (2002). *Promoting Women's Health A population investment for Ireland's future*. The Women's Health Council: Dublin.

WHO. (2000). World Health Organization: Guiding principles for feeding infants and young children in emergencies. *The Management of Nutrition in Major Emergencies, Annex 5, 202–203, Annex 6*, pp 207–212. 588–590.

WHO. (2001). World Health Organization: Expert Consultation on the Optimal Duration of Exclusive Breastfeeding. WHO, Geneva Switzerland: WHO reference number: WHO/NHD/01.09, WHO/FCH/CAH/01.24.

WHO. (2003). Guiding principles for feeding infants and young children during emergencies. Department of Nutrition for Health and Development, WHO: Geneva.

WHO/UNICEF. (1989). Protecting, Promoting and Supporting Breastfeeding – The special role of the maternity services. A Joint WHO/UNICEF Statement: Geneva.

WHO/UNICEF. (1997). HIV and Infant feeding. A policy statement developed collaboratively by UNAIDS, WHO and UNICEF: Geneva.

WHO/UNICEF. (2002). *Global Strategy for Infant and Young Child Feeding*. World Health Organization: Geneva.

Williamson, J. and Moser, A. (1988). *Unaccompanied Children in Emergencies: a Field Guide for Their Care and Protection*. Geneva, Switzerland: International Social Service.

Woolridge, M.W. (1995). Baby-controlled breastfeeding: Bio-cultural implications. In: *Breastfeeding: Bio-cultural perspectives. P. Stuart-Macadam and KA Dettwyler* (eds). New York: Aldine de Gruyter.

World Health Organization. (1981). *International code of marketing of breast-milk substitutes*. Geneva.

World Health Organization. (1998). Relactation: A review of experience and recommendations for practice. Retrieved on 12-11-2008 from

http://www.who.int/child-adolescent-
health/publications/NUTRITION/WHO_CHS_CAH_98.14.htm.

Yip, R. and Sharp, T.W. (1993). Acute malnutrition and high childhood mortality related to diarrhea: lessons from the 1991 Kurdish refugee crisis. *JAMA,* 270, 587-90.

Zinn B. (2000). Supporting the employed breastfeeding mother. *Journal of Midwifery and Women's Health*, 45, 216-26.

INDEX

K

L

Q

R

S

self-confidence, 101
seminars, 82, 83
sensing, 51
sensitivity, 34, 52
sensitization, ix, 42, 43, 52, 59, 61, 68
serotonin, 5
serum, 19, 51
services, iv, 102, 112, 130
sex, 10, 17
sex hormones, 17
sex steroid, 10
showing, 22, 47, 51, 53, 60, 62
siblings, 44, 46
signals, 57
signs, 18, 33, 36, 38, 77
Sinai, 10
skeletal muscle, 50
skin, 57, 69, 110
small intestine, 56
SNP, 3
social attitudes, 8
social context, 92
social environment, 113
social influence, 78
social learning, 78
social learning theory, 78
social status, 113
social support, 115
society, 38, 101, 113
South Africa, 126
Soviet Union, 103
Spain, 5, 41, 64
spasticity, vii, 2, 4, 6
specialists, 109
species, 44, 45, 46, 54, 67
spontaneous abortion, viii, 16, 20
storage, 50, 65, 96
stress, x, 50, 69, 93, 96, 97, 103, 106, 108
stretching, 122
style, 83
subgroups, 63, 84
substitutes, 106, 108, 109, 110, 111, 114, 130
substrates, 20
succession, ix, 42, 43, 44

Sudan, 99, 100, 103, 128
sudden infant death syndrome, 96, 102
Sudden Infant Death Syndrome, 129
supervision, 115
supplementation, 43, 55, 56, 57, 61, 62, 63, 68, 109
suppression, 3
surface area, 48
surgical intervention, 36
surveillance, 6
survey, 7, 12, 66, 76, 92, 93, 99, 100, 116, 119, 120, 123
survival, 43, 96, 100, 109
susceptibility, ix, 3, 9, 42, 43
Sweden, 5, 75
Switzerland, 130
symptoms, vii, 2, 5, 6, 18, 20, 21, 33, 36
syndrome, 19, 26, 96, 102
synthesis, 49

T

T cell, 4, 10, 51, 52, 57, 62, 67
tachycardia, 33
Taiwan, 124
target, 78, 101, 113
teacher training, 114
techniques, 12, 20
temperature, 34
testing, 21
testosterone, 19
tetanus, 106
TF, 37
TGF, 3, 52, 59, 61
therapy, 11, 13, 36
threonine, 49
thyroid, 16
TLR, 51, 57
TLR2, 52, 57
TLR4, 57
TLR9, 69
TNF, 51, 56, 59, 60
TNF-α, 51
toddlers, 100
Togo, 116
trade, 99